MEDICAL HIEROGLYPHS

Abbreviations and Symbols

Avice H. Kerr R.N., B.A.

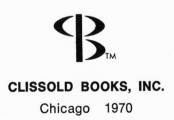

CLISSOLD BOOKS, INC.

Chicago 1970

Author's Preface

These symbols and abbreviations have been taken from medical records and the meanings obtained from the persons who used them.

Not all of these abbreviations are formally recognized by hospital committees who decide such things but for those of us who must transcribe hand written notes from doctor's offices as well as hospitals, it is of little value to know that an abbreviation is "not recognized" since the doctor will use it anyhow. We can only learn the meaning it is intended to convey.

Since one abbreviation may mean many things, it is necessary to know enough about the context to select the meaning intended.

I would like to express my appreciation to all those secretaries who, in turn, worked on this material even though they disliked doing this kind of detail. But my special gratitude goes to my daughter, Lynne Boozel, who with infinite patience rearranged and retyped these listings many times. Without her work on this manuscript, done as a labor of love, this book would not now be available.

MEDICAL HIEROGLYPHS

Abbreviations

MEDICAL HIEROGLYPHS

Abbreviations

A	accommodation
A *acetum*	dilution in acetic acid
A	acid
A	(total) acidity
A	actin
A	action, active, activity
A	allergist, allergy
A	alpha
A	amphere
A *annum*	year
A	anode
A	answer
A *ante*	before
A	anterior
A	aorta
A *aqua*	water
A	aqueous
A	area
A	argon

A	artery
A	asymmetric, asymmetry
A	atria
A	atrophy
A	axial
A	axilla, axillary
Å, Å	Angstrom unit
A#1, A#2, etc.	auto number one, auto number 2 (in description of traffic accident)
a	action, active, activity
a	ampere
a *ante*	before
a	level of significance
a* Greek letter alpha	1) in proportion to 2) first (in organic compounds refers to the carbon atom which follows next to carbon atom bearing the active group of molecule)
@	at
AA	Achievement Age
AA	active assisted (exercises)
AA	Alcoholics Anonymous
AA *ana*	equal parts, of each
AA	Associate in Arts (Degree obtained on completion of a prescribed course in a two year college)
AA	atlantoaxial, atloaxoid

* Included here because when handwritten alpha often looks like an a

AA	auto accident
ā̄ā, ā̄ā, ȧȧ *ana*	equal parts, of each
aaa	amalgam
AABS	auto accident, broadside
AAE, AA ex	active assisted exercises
AAF	acetic-alcohol-formalin
AAF	ascorbic acid factor
AAGP	American Academy of General Practice
AAL	anterior axillary line
AAMC	Association of American Medical Colleges
AAMIH	American Association for Maternal and Infant Health
AAMRL	American Association of Medical Records Librarians (This name has now been changed — see AMRA)
AAO	awake, alert and oriented (state of consciousness)
AAO	American Association of Orthodontists
AAOP	American Academy of Oral Pathology
AAP	American Academy of Pediatricians
AAP	American Academy of Peridontology
AARE	auto accident, rear end
AB	abortion
AB	Ace bandage Example: AB→ rt leg, toes→↑ thigh = Ace bandage to right leg, toes to upper thigh
AB	active bilaterally (reflexes)

AB	Aid to the Blind
AB	Bachelor of Arts
AB	antibodies
AB	asthmatic bronchitis
AB	axiobuccal (planes of tooth)
Ab	abortion
Ab	alabamine
Ab	antibodies
ab	abortion
ab	about
abbr, abbrev	abbreviated, abbreviation
ABC	atomic, biological and chemical (warfare)
ABC	axiobuccocervical (planes of tooth)
A ∉ BC	air and bone conduction (hearing)
ABD (pad)	abdominal pad (a large absorbent pad which is placed over abdominal dressings)
Abd, abd	abdomen, abdominal
abd	abduct, abduction (to move away from the midline of the body)
abd	abductor (muscles which move an extremity away from the midline of the body)
abdo, abdom	abdomen, abdominal
aber	aberrant, aberration
ABG	axiobuccogingival (planes of tooth)
ABL	axiobuccolingual (planes of tooth)
abn, abnor, abnorm	abnormal, abnormality

ABO	absent bed occupant (patient out on leave)
ABP	arterial blood pressure
ABPS θ	albumin, blood, pus and sugar negative (urinalysis)
ABR	absolute bed rest
abr, abras	abrasion
ABS	acute brain syndrome
abs	absent
abs	absolute
absc	abscess
abs feb *abstante febre*	absence of fever
abs fev *abstante fevre*	absence of fever
AbSR	abdominal skin reflexes
abst, abstr	abstract
abt	about
AC	acromioclavicular
AC	adrenal cortex
AC	air conduction (hearing)
AC	alternating current
AC	anodal closure
AC *ante cibum*	before meals
AC	anterior chamber (eye)
AC	antiphlogistic corticoid
AC	atriocarotid

AC	auriculocarotid
AC	axiocervical
A/C	acromioclavicular
Ac	acceleration
Ac	acetyl
Ac	acid carbonate (H_2CO_3)
Ac	actinium
Ac	acute
Ac	anodal closure
ac	acceleration
ac	acute
ac, a/c	alternating current
ac	anodal closure
ac	anterior chamber (eye)
ACA	anterior cerebral artery
ACA	anterior coronary artery
ACA	anterior communicating aneurysms
acad	academy
AC/BC	air conduction time/bone conduction time
ACC	anodal closing contraction
Acc	acceleration, accelerator
acc	accident
acc	accommodation
acc	accompany
acc	according

accel	accelerate, accelerated, acceleration
Ac Ch	acetylcholine
accid	accident, accidental
acc insuff	accomodative insufficiency (eyes)
ACCL, ACCl	anodal closure clonus
Ac Co A	acetyl coenzyme A
accom	accommodation (eye)
accom	accompanied, accompany
accum	accumulate, accumulated, accumulative
ACD	absolute cardiac dullness
ACD sol	citric acid, trisodium citrate, dextrose solution
ace	acetone
ACE	adrenocortical extract
ACE bandage	This is not an abbreviation but the trade name of a type of elastic bandage
ACE mix	alcohol, chloroform, ether mixture
AC Em	actinium emanation (actinon)
acet	acetone
acetab	acetabulum
ACF	accessory clinical findings
ACG	angiocardiography
ACH	adrenocortical hormone
ACh	acetylcholine
ā ch ā	as much as
AChE	acetylcholinesterase

ACH index	arm, chest hip index (Index of nutrition based on circumferential measurements of arms, depth of chest and hip width)
A C hyph	anterior chamber hyphemia
ACI	acute coronary insufficiency
acid p'tase	acid phosphatase
AC jt	acromioclavicular joint
ACL	anterior clavicular line
ACO	alert, cooperative and oriented (description of state of consciousness)
ACO	anodal closing odor
ACP	American College of Physicians
ACP	anodal closing picture
ACPP	adrenocorticopolypeptide
ACR	American College of Radiology
ACR	anticonstipation regime
A/C ratio	albumin coagulin ratio
ACS	American College of Surgeons
ACS	anodal closing sound
ACS	antiventricular cytotoxic serum
act	action, active, activity
=/act, =$\notin$ act	equal and active (pupils, deep tendon reflexes)
ACTe	anodal closing tetanus
ACTH	adrenocorticotrophic hormone
ACTP	adrenocorticotrophic polypeptide
ACTS	acute cervical traumatic sprain

ACTS	acute cervical traumatic syndrome
ACTS c̄ NRI	acute cervical traumatic syndrome with nerve root involvement
AD	adenoidal degeneration
AD	adult disease
AD	anodal duration
AD *atrio dextro*	right atrium
AD *auris dextra*	right ear
AD	average deviation
AD	axiodistal
AD	diphenylchlorarsine
A ∉ D	admission and discharge
ad *adde*	let it be added (pharmacy)
ad	axiodistal
ADA	American Diabetic Association
ADA	American Dietetic Association
ADA	American Dental Association
ADC	Aid to Dependent Children
ADC-U	Aid to Dependent Children of Unemployed
AD capacity	alveolar diffusing capacity
ADC	anodal duration contraction
ADC	axiodistocervical
add *adde*	let it be added (pharmacy)

add	added, additional, addition
add	adduct, adduction (to move toward the midline of the body)
add	adductor (muscles that move an extremity toward the midline of the body)
ad def an *ad defectionem animi*	to the point of fainting
ad deliq *ad deliquium*	to the point of fainting
addict	addiction
addn	addition
addnl	additional
ad duas vic *ad duas vices*	to two doses, for two doses
ad effect *ad effectum*	until effectual
adeq	adequate
ad feb *adstante febre*	having fever
ad fev *adstante fevre*	having fever
ADG	axiodistogingival (planes of tooth)
ad gr acid, ad grat acid *ad gratum aciditatem*	to an agreeable acidity
ad gr gust, ad grat gust *ad gratum gustum*	to an agreeable taste
ADH	antidiuretic hormone (vasopressin)
adh	adhesions
adh	adhesive
adhes	adhesions

adhes	adhesive
adhib *adhibendus*	to be administered
ADI	axiodistoincisal
ADI	axiodistoinclusal
ad int *ad interim*	in the meantime, in the interim
adj	adjacent
adj	adjoining
adj	adjunct
adj	adjust, adjusted
Adj. Of.	Adjudication Office (or officer)
ADL	activities of daily living
ad lib *ad libitum*	as desired, freely
ADM	Administrative Medicine
Adm	administration, administrator
adm	admission, admit, admitted
adm amb	admitted ambulatory
Adm Dr	admitting doctor
admin	administer, administration
Adm Ph, Adm Phys	admitting physician
adm w/c	admitted in wheelchair
admov *admoveatur*	let it be applied, apply
ad neut *ad neutro*	neutralize, neutralized, neutralization

ADO   axiodisto-occlusal (planes of tooth)

ADP   automatic data processing

ad part dol   to the painful part
  ad parte dolente

ADPL   average daily patient load

ad pond om   to the weight of the whole
  ad pondus omnium

ADR   Accepted Dental Remedies

Adr, adr   adrenalin

ad rat   to ratio (pharmacy)
  ad rationem

adren   adrenalin

ADS   antidiuretic substance

ad sat   to saturation
  ad saturandum

Adson's M   Adson's maneuver

adst feb   when fever is present
  adstante febre

adst fev   when fever is present
  adstante fevre

ADT   any desired thing (placebo)

ADT   adenosine triphosphate

ADTe   anodal duration tetanus

ad tert vic   for three doses, three times
  ad tertium vicem

ad us   according to custom, according to usage
  ad usum

ad us ext   for external use
  ad usum externum

ad us propr *ad usum proprium*	according to proper use
adv *adversum*	against
adv	advice, advise
ADW	assault with a deadly weapon
AE	above elbow
A ¢ E	active and equal
ae *aetatis*	at age of, of age
AE amp	above elbow amputation
AEC	at earliest convenience
AEC	Atomic Energy Commission
aeg *aegra*	patient
A Eq	age equivalent
aeq *aequales*	equal
Aero, aero	aerobacter (bacteria which grows where air is present)
AES	American Encephalographic Society
AES	American Epidemiological Society
aet, aetat *aetatis*	at age of, of age
AF	acid fast
AF	adult female
AF	Air Force
AF	Armed Forces

AF	Arthritis Foundation
AF	atrial fibrillation
AF	audio frequency
AF	auricular fibrillation
AFB	acid fast bacilli
AFB	Air Force Base
AFB	American Foundation for the Blind
AFDC	Aid to Families of Dependent Children
afeb	afebrile
aff	afferent
aff *affinis*	affinity
affil	affiliated
AFIP	Armed Forces Institute of Pathology
AFL	artificial limb
AFML	Armed Forces Medical Library
AfP, Af Ph	affiliate Physician
AFTR	atrophy, fasciculation, tremor, rigidity
AG	antigravity, against gravity
AG	atrial gallop
AG, A/G (ratio)	albumin-globulin ratio
AG, A/G (suit)	antigravity suit (used in medicine to control shock by external pressure)
AG	axiogingival
Ag	antigen

Ag *argentum*	silver
ag	antigravity
ag	atrial gallop
AGA	accelerated growth area (embryology)
AGB, agb	any good brand
Ag Cl$_2$	silver chloride
AGCT	Army General Classification Test
Agcy, agcy	agency
AGE, ÅGE, A° GE	angle of greatest extension
AGF, ÅGF, A° GF	angle of greatest flexion
ag feb *aggrediente febre*	when fever increases, increasing fever
ag fev *aggrediente fevre*	when fever increases, increasing fever
agg, aggl, agglut	agglutinate, agglutination
aggrav	aggravate, aggravation
agit *agita*	shake, stir (pharmacy)
agit	agitated, agitation (psychology or psychiatry)
agit ante sum *agita ante sumedum*	shake before taking
agit a us *agita ante usum*	shake before using
agit bene *agite bene*	shake well
agit vas *agite vase*	shake the vial
AGN	albumin globulin studies

agn	agnosia
AgNO$_3$	silver nitrate
agt	agent
AGV	anilin gentian violet
ah, a h	ampere hour
A ₵ H ins	accident and health insurance
AH, ah	hypermetropic astigmatism, hyperopic astigmatism
AHA	American Heart Association
AHA	American Hospital Association
AHD	acute heart disease
AHD	auto-immune hemolytic disease
AHF	American Hospital Formulary
AHF	antihemolytic factor (factor viii)
AHF	antihemophilic factor
AHG	antihemophilic globulin
AHG	antihemolytic globulin, antihemolytic globulin factor (factor viii)
AHG	antihuman globulin
AHN	Assistant Head Nurse
AI	accidentally incurred
AI	aortic insufficiency
AI	apical impulse
AI	artificial insemination
AI	axioincisal (planes of tooth)
A/I, ai	accidentally incurred

AIBS	American Institute of Biological Sciences
AID	acute infectious disease
AID	artificial insemination by donor
AIH	artificial insemination by husband
AIIS	anterior inferior iliac spine
A insuf	aortic insufficiency
AIP	anatuberculin, Petragnanis' integral
Air Bronch	air bronchogram
AIT	acute intensive treatment
AJ	ankle jerk
AK	above knee
A→K	ankle to knee
AKA	also known as
AK amp	above knee amputation
AL	adaptation level
AL	alignment mark (cardiography)
AL	axilla loop
AL	axiolingual (tooth planes)
Al	aluminum
al	alignment
al	alignment mark (cardiography)
A La	axiolabial (tooth planes)
A La L	axiolabiolingual (tooth planes)
Alb, alb	albumin
alb C	albumin clearance

ALC	avian leukosis complex
ALC	axiolinguocervical (tooth planes)
Alc, alc, alcoh	alcohol, alcoholic
Alc R	alcohol rub
ALG	axiolinguogingival (planes of tooth)
alg, algy	allergy
ALH	anterior lobe hypophysis
align	alignment
aliq *aliquot*	some, several
alk	alkaline
alk phos, alk p'tase	alkaline phosphatase
ALL	acute lymphatic leukemia
ALL	allergy
alleg	alleged, allegedly
ALO	axiolinguoclusal (tooth planes)
ALR	Ear, Nose and Throat (designation of medical specialty of Otology, Laryngology and Rhinology)
ALS	amyotrophic lateral sclerosis
alt	alternate
alt	altitude
alt die, alt dieb *alternis diebus*	alternate days, every other day
alt h, alt hor *alternis horis*	alternate hours, every other hour
alt noc, alt noct *alternis nocte*	alternate nights, every other night

ALTS	acute lumbar traumatic sprain
ALTS	acute lumbar traumatic syndrome
alv	alveolar
alv vent	alveolar ventilation
alv adst *alvi adstricta*	constipated
Alv-Art, alv-art	alveolar-arterial difference
alv deject *alvi dejectiones*	alvine dejections (intestinal waste, feces)
Alv PO_2, alv PO_2	alveolar oxygen pressure
ALVF	acute left ventricular failure
ALW	arch-loop-whorl
AM	actomycin
AM	adult male
AM	ampere meter
AM	amplitude modulation
AM *ante meridian*	before noon
AM	articular manipulation
AM *Artium Magister*	Master of Arts
AM (prosthesis)	Austin-Moore prosthesis
AM	Aviation Medicine (designation of medical specialty – a special field of Preventive Medicine)
AM	axiomesial (tooth planes)
AM	meter angle
AM	myopic astigmatism

A/M	adult male
A-M	Austin-Moore prosthesis
Am	american
Am	americium
A/m	amperes per minute
am	ametropia
am	ammeter
am	ampere minute
am	amyl
am	myopic astigmatism
AMA	against medical advice
AMA	American Medical Association
ama	against medical advice
ama, áṁà, a̅m̅a̅	as much as, as many as
AMAL	AeroMedical Acceleration Laboratory
amb	ambulance
amb	ambulate, ambulation, ambulatory Example: amb PWB lft 20# = ambulatory partial weight bearing on the left with maximum pressure of 20 pounds
ambig	ambiguous
ambul	ambulate, ambulatory, ambulation
AMC	axiomesiocervical (tooth planes)
Am ₵ Ct	antibiotic medical and clinical therapy
AMD	axiomesiodistal (tooth planes)
AMEDS	Army Medical Corps
Amer, amer	american

AMG	axiomesiogingival
AMH, Am h	mixed astigmatism with exceeding myopia, mixed astigmatism with marked myopia
AMI	acute myocardial infarction
AMI	axiomesioincisal
ammon	ammonia
amor, amorph	amorphous
AMP	adenosine monophosphate
amp	ampere, amperage
amp	amplitude
amp	ampule
amp	amputate, amputated, amputation
amph	amphoric
amp-hr	ampere hour
ampl	amplitude
A-M prosthesis	Austin-Moore prosthesis
ampt	amputation, amputee
AMR	alternate motion rate
AMRA	American Medical Records Association
AMS	auditory memory span
AMSC	Army Medical Specialist Corps
AMT	American Medical Technologists
amt	amount
AMU, amu	atomic mass unit
AMVET	American Veteran World War II

amyl	amylase
AN	normal atmosphere
An	actinon
An	anisometropia
An	anodal, anode
An	normal atmosphere
ANA	American Nurse's Association
anal	analgesia, analgesic
Anal	analysis, analyze
Anal Psych	Analytical Psychology
anat	anatomic, anatomical, anatomy
ant align	anatomical alignment
ANC	Army Nurse Corps
AnCC	anodal closure contraction
An D Te	anodal duration tetanus
Anaes, anes, anesth	anesthesia, anesthesiologist, anesthetic, anesthesiology
an ex	anodal excitation
ANF	antinuclear factor
Ang, ang	angle, angulation
ang pect	angina pectoris
anh, anhyd	anhydrous
ANI	acute nerve irritation
ann	annals
AnOc	anodal opening contraction

ANRI	acute nerve root irritation
ANS	autonomic nervous system
ans	answer
ANT *2-amino-5-nitrothiazol*	Enheptin
ant	anterior
antag	antagonism, antagonistic
ant ax	anterior axillary line
ante (Not an abbreviation)	a prefix meaning before
anthro	anthropologist, anthropology
anthropom	anthropometry
ant jentac *ante jentaculum*	before breakfast (pharmacy)
ant long ligs	anterior longitudinal ligaments
ant pit	anterior pituitary
ant prand *ante prandium*	before dinner (pharmacy)
ant sup sp	anterior superior spine
ant tib	anterior tibial
ANTU	alphanaphthylthiourea
anx	anxiety, anxious
AO	anodal opening
AO	atrioventricular (valve) opening
Ao	aorta
ao, a/o	angle of
AOC	anodal opening contraction

AOCl	anodal opening clonus
AOD	arteriosclerotic occlusive disease
AO diag	acridine-orange diagnosis
AOM *Artium Obstetricus Magister*	Master of Obstetric Art
AOO	anodal opening odor
AOP	anodal opening picture
aort regurg	aortic regurgitation
aort sten	aortic stenosis
AOS	anodal opening sound
AOTA	American Occupational Therapists Association
AOTe	anodal opening tetanus
AO tech	acridine-orange technic (a 2 color fluorescence test)
AOW	admitted from other ward
AP	action potential
AP	after parturition
AP	alum precipitated
AP *ante prandium*	before dinner (pharmacy)
AP	anterior pituitary
AP	anteroposterior
AP	aortic pressure
AP	aortic pulmonary
AP *apriori*	prior to
AP	apical pulse

AP	axiopulpal (planes of tooth)
A-P	alum precipitated
A-P	aortic-pulmonary
Ap, ap	apothecary
3 AP	3-acetylpyridine
↑AP	anteroposterior (chest) measurement increased
↓AP	anteroposterior (chest) measurement decreased
A ∉ P	active and present (reflexes)
A ∉ P	anatomy and physiology
A ∉ P	anterior and posterior
A ∉ P	auscultation and percussion
$A_2 > P_2$	aortic second sound greater than pulmonary second sound
$A_2 = P_2$	aortic second sound equals pulmonary second sound
$A_2 < P_2$	aortic second sound less than pulmonary second sound
APA	action potential amplitude
APA	American Physiotherapy Association
APA	American Psychiatric Association
APAF	antipernicious anemia factor
APC	aspirin, phenacetin and caffeine compound
APC	atrial premature contractions
APC virus	adenoidal, pharyngeal and conjunctival virus
APD	action potential duration
APE	anterior pituitary extract

APF	animal protein factor
APH	anterior pituitary hormone
aph	aphasia
APL	anterior pituitary-like substance
AP ∉ L, AP ∉ Lat	anteroposterior and lateral (xray views)
APM	alternating pressure mattress
apoth	apothecary
app	apparatus
app	apparent, apparently
app	appears
app	appendix
app	appointment
app	appropriate
appar	apparatus
appl	application
appl	applied
appl	appliance
applan *applanatus*	flattened
applic	application
appoint	appointment
appos	apposition (contact of two surfaces)
Apoth, apoth	apothecary
appr, approx	approximate, approximately
appt	appointment

appy	appendectomy
APR	anterior pituitary reaction
APR	anterior primary rami
apr	apraxia
APS	adenosine phosphosulfate
APT	aluminum precipitated toxoid
AQ	accomplishment quotient
AQ	achievement quotient
aq *aqua*	aqueous, water
aq astr *aqua astricta*	frozen water
Aq bul *aqua bulliens*	boiling water
aq comm *aqua communis*	common water
aq dist *aqua distilla*	distilled water
aq ferv *aqua fervens*	hot water
aq fluv *aqua fluvalis*	river water
aq font *aqua fontana*	spring water
aq mar *aqua marina*	sea water
aq niv *aqua nivalis*	snow water
aq pen	aqueous penicillin

aq pluv *aqua pluvialis*	rain water
aq pur *aqua pura*	pure water
aq tep *aqua tepid*	tepid (lukewarm) water
aqu	aqueous
AR	achievement ratio
AR	active resistive (exercises)
AR	Admitting Room
AR	alarm reaction
AR	analytical reagent
AR	apical rate
AR	arsphenamine
AR	auricular rate
A/R, A-R	apical-radial
A-R	active resistive (exercises)
ar	argon
ARC	anomalous retinal correspondence
Arch, arch	archives
ARD	absolute reaction of degeneration
ARD	acute respiratory disease
ARD	all related data
ARD	ano-rectal dressing
ARDC	Air research and Development Command
ARE	active-resistive exercises

ARF	Arthritis and Rheumatism Foundation (now Arthritis Foundation)
arg *argentum*	silver
Arg-Rob	Argyll-Robertson Symptoms
ARI	anxiety reaction, intense
ARM	anxiety reaction, mild
ARM	artificial rupture of membranes (obstetrics)
AROM	active range of motion
arom	aromatic
ARP	absolute refractory period
ARPT	American Registry of Physical Therapists
A-R pulse	apical-radial pulse
arr	arrested (status of disease)
Ars	arsphenamine
ART	Accredited Record Technician
Art, art	arterial, artery
art	artificial
arth	arthritic, arthritis
arthrot	arthrotomy
artic	articular, articulation
artic manip	articular manipulation
artif	artificial
art insem	artificial insemination
Art PO_2, art PO_2	arterial oxygen pressure
AS	anal sphincter

AS	aortic sounds
AS	aortic stenosis
AS	aqueous solution
AS	aqueous suspension
AS	arteriosclerosis
AS	ascendence submission
AS	astigmatism
AS *auris sininster*	left ear
A-S (syndrome)	Adams-Stokes syndrome
A-S	arteriosclerosis
A-S	ascendence submission
As	arsenic
As, as	astigmatism
ASA	acetylsalicylic acid (aspirin)
ASA	American Society of Anesthesiologists
ASA	American Standards Association
ASA, āsā, aṡa	as soon as
ASAP	as soon as possible
ASC	ascorbic acid
ASC, asc	arteriosclerosis
ASCP	American Society of Clinical Pathologists
ascr *ascriptum*	ascribe to
ASCVD, AS & CVD	aeteriosclerotic cardiovascular disease
ASD	atrio-septal defect

asex	asexual
A ¢ SH, a ¢ sh	arm and shoulder
AsH	hyperopic (hypermetropic) astigmatism
ASHD	arteriosclerotic heart disease
ASHD	atrioseptal heart defect
ASIS	anterior superior iliac spine
ASIS→IM	anterior superior iliac spine to internal malleolus
ASIS→MM	anterior superior iliac spine to medial malleolus
ASL	antistreptolysin (titer)
AsM	myopic astigmatism
ASO	antistreptolysin O (titer)
ASO	arteriosclerosis obliterans
asp	aspect
asp	aspirate, aspirated, aspiration
ASS	anterior superior spine
assim	assimilate, assimilated
assist	assistance, assistant
Assn, assn	association
assoc	associate, associated, association
assoc'd	associated
asst	assist
AST	antistreptolysin test (for ACTH tolerance)
AST	antistreptolysin titer
Ast	astigmatism
A sten	aortic stenosis

asth	asthenia
asth	asthenopia
asth	asthma
as tol	as tolerated
asw	artificially sweetened
asx	asymptomatic
asym	asymmetrical
AT	achievement test
AT	adjunctive therapy
AT	air temperature
AT	air tight
AT *alt tuberculin*	old tuberculin
AT	anterior tibial (pulse)
AT *tibialis anticus*	name of muscle, lateral tibial surface
AT	dihydrotachysterol
At	astatine
at	additional term (different name for the same disease) synonym, eponym
at	air tight
at	ampere turn
at	atom, atomic
ATHF	allotetrahydrocortisol
athsc	atherosclerosis
atm, atmos	atmosphere, atmospheric

at no	atomic number
ATP	adenosine triphosphate
At P'ase	adenosine triphosphatase
ATPD	ambient temperature and pressure, dry
At P, At Phys	Attending Physician
ATPS	ambient temperature and pressure, saturated
ATR	achilles tendon reflex
atr	atrophy
atrop	atropine
ATS	antitetanic serum
ATS	anxiety tension state
AT type	Adenine and Thymine type
at vol	atomic volume
at wt	atomic weight
atyp	atypical
AU	Angstrom unit
AU	antitoxin unit (diphtheria)
AU *auris unitas*	both ears
Au *aurum*	gold
aud	auditory
aur	auricle, auricular
aur *aures*	ears
aur *auris*	ear

aur fib	auricular fibrillation
auric	auricle, auricular
aus	auscultation
auscul	auscultation
aux	auxillary
AV	air velocity
AV	arteriovascular
AV	arteriovenous
AV (nicking)	arteriovenous nicking
AV (ratio)	arteriovenous ratio
AV	atrioventricular
AV	augmented vector
AV	auriculoventricular
A-V	arterio-venous
Av	air velocity
av	arterio-venous
av	average
av	avoirdupois
av	avulsion
AVA	arteriovascular anastomosis
avdp	avoirdupois
aver	average
AVF, aVF	left foot lead in electrocardiogram
av fx	avulsion fracture
avg	average

AVL, aVL	left arm lead in electrocardiogram
AVO	atrioventricular opening
avoir	avoirdupois
AVR, aVR	right arm lead in electrocardiogram
AV shunt	arteriovenous shunt
AW	aluminum wafer
A ∉ W	active and well
A ∉ W	alive and well
A/W	able to work
awa, åẘå, ā̄w̄ā	as well as
AWDW	assault with a deadly weapon
AWF	adrenal weight factor
AWL	absent with leave (i.e. permitted to leave the hospital for a specified period)
AWOL	absent without leave
AWRU	active wrist rotation unit
ax	axial
ax	axilla, axillary
ax	axis
ax grad	axial gradient
Az azote	nitrogen
az	azobacter
AZT	Ascheim-Zondek test (for pregnancy)

B	bacillus
B	barometric
B	base
B	bath
B	Baumé scale
B	behavior
B	Benoist scale
B	bicuspid
B	bipass or shunt
B	body (in psychiatry, all the body except the nervous system)
B	born
B	boron
B	brother
B	buccal
B *bis*	twice
B	gauss
b	bacillus
b *bis*	twice
b	boils at
b	born
B_6	pyridoxine
BA	Bachelor of Arts
BA	backache

BA	basilar artery
BA	blood alchohol
BA	boric acid
BA	brachial artery
BA	bronchial asthma
BA	buccoaxial
B/A	backache
Ba	barium
B ∉ A	brisk and active (reflexes)
BAA	benzoyl arginine amide
Bab	Babinski's reflex, Babinski's sign
BAC	bacterial antigen complex
BAC	buccoaxiocervical (tooth planes)
bac	bacillus
$BaCl_2$, BaCl	barium chloride
bact	bacteria, bacterial, bacteriology
bacti	bacteriology
BaE, BaEn, Ba Enem	barium enema
BAG	buccoaxiogingival (tooth planes)
BAI	basilar artery insufficiency
BAIB	beta aminoisobutyric acid
BAL	British antilewisite (used in arsenic poisoning) dimercaprol
bal	balance
bals	balsam

BAO	Bachelor of Arts of Obstetrics
bapt	baptized
bar	barometer, barometric
Barb, barb	barbiturate
BAS	benzyl analog of serotonin
bas	basilar
baso	basophil, basophilic
Ba sol	boric acid solution
basos	basophils
BB	bed boards
BB	Bellevue bridge — an adhesive bridge from thigh to thigh to elevate the scrotum
BB	both bones (of arm or leg)
BB	buffer base
bb	ball bearing
bb	bed boards
bb	both bones (of arm or leg)
BBA	born before arrival
BBB	blood-brain barrier
BBB	bundle branch block (heart)
BBC	brombenzylcyanide
B bridge	Bellevue bridge (scrotal support)
BBT	basal body temperature
BC	Bachelor of Chemistry
BC	bone conduction (hearing)

BC	buccocervical (tooth planes)
B/C, B ₵ C	breathed and cried (newborn infant)
BC_{51}	cholinesterase inhibitor
bc	back care
b/c	because
b/c, b ₵ c	breathed and cried
BCD	Bad Conduct Discharge (U.S. Army)
BCG	Bacillus Calmette Guerin (vaccine for tuberculosis)
BCG	ballistocardiogram
BCG	bromcresyl green
BCG (test)	bicolor guiac test
BCH	basal cell hyperplasia
B CH *Chirurgiae Baccalaureus*	Bachelor of Surgery
B comp	(vitamin) B complex
BCP	birth control pills
BCP	bromcresyl purple
BCR	birth control regime
BCRx, BCR	birth control treatment, birth control medication
BD	base of prism down
BD	Baudelocque's diameter
BD	birth date
BD	buccodistal (tooth planes)
bd	board

bd *bis die*	twice daily
BDB	bisdiazotized benzidine
BDS	Bachelor of Dental Surgery
BDSc	Bachelor of Dental Science
BE	bacillen emulsion
BE	barium enema
BE	base excess (negative indicates deficit)
BE	below elbow
B↓E	both lower extremities
B↑E	both upper extremities
B ≸ E	brisk and equal (equal)
Bé	Baumé (specific gravity scale)
Be	beryllium
BEA, Be amp	below elbow amputation
bef	before
beg	began, begin, beginning
beh	behavior, behaviorism
BEI	serum butanol-extractable iodine
bellig	belligerent
benz	benzidine
benz	benzoate
Benz test	benzidine test (to determine presence of blood)
bet	between
bev	beverage

bev	billion electron volts
BF	body fat
BF	boullon filtre (Deny's tuberculin)
BFO	balanced forearm orthesis
BFP	biological false positive (reaction)
BFR sol	buffered Ringer's solution
BFS	blood fasting sugar (rarely used – usually written FBS)
BFT	bentonite flocculation test
BG	Bordet-Gengou (bacillus)
BG	buccogingival
B-G	Bordet-Gengou bacillus
b/g	began
BGLB	brilliant green lactose broth
BGS	balance, gait, station
BHA	bilateral hilar adenopathy
BHC	benzene hexachloride
BHIB	beef heart infusion broth
BHL	biological half life
BHN	Brinell hardness number
BHP	benign hypertrophic prostatitis
BI	base of prism in
BI, B-I	bi-ischial (obstetric pelvimetry)
BI, B/I	body injury
Bi	biceps

Bi	bismuth
BIB	brought in by (Emergency Room or hospital admission record)
bib *bibe*	drink
biblio, bibliog	bibliography
bic	biceps
bicarb	sodium bicarbonate
BID, bid *bis in die*	twice in a day
bigem	bigeminy (the occurence of two beats of the heart in rapid succession)
bihor *bihorium*	during two hours
Bi Isch, bi isch	between the ischial tuberosities
BIL	brother-in-law
bil	bilateral
bil	bilirubin
bilat	bilateral
bili	bilirubin
BIN *bis in noct*	twice during the night
biochem	biochemist, biochemistry
bioeng	bioengineering
biol	biological, biologist, biology
BIP	bacterial intravenous protein
BIP	bismuth iodoform petrolatum, bismuth iodoform paraffin

BIPP	bismuth iodoform petrolatum paste
Bird	Bird respirator
Bi sp	between ischial spines
BIT, Bi T, bitroch	bitrochanteric
BIW, biw	twice a week
BJ	biceps jerk
B/J, B ₵ J	bone and joint
BK	below knee
Bk amp	below knee amputation
Bk	berkelium
bk	back
bkd	baked
bkly	backlying
BL *balneum luteum*	mud bath
BL	blood loss
BL	body lean
BL	buccolingual (tooth planes)
Bl	base balanced carbonate
bl	bleeding
bl	blood
bl	black
bl ₵ blue	black and blue
bl cult	blood culture
Bld, bld	blood

Bld Bnk	Blood Bank
BLE	both lower extremities
blk	black
BL min	blood loss minimal
BLQ	both lower quadrants
Bl T	blood test
Bl vol	blood volume
BM	Bachelor of Medicine
BM *balneum maris*	sea water bath
BM	basal metabolism
BM	basement membrane
BM	bowel movement
BM	buccomesial
BMR	basal metabolism rate
BMS	Bachelor of Medical Science
BNA *Basle Nomina Anatomica*	basal anatomical nomenclature
BND	barely noticeable difference
BNO	bladder neck obstruction
BO	base of prism out
BO	body odor
BO	buccoclusal (tooth planes)
B ∉ O	belladonna and opium
bo	bowel
BOA	born out of asepsis

BOD	biochemical oxygen demand
Bod U	Bodansky unit (with reference to alkaline phosphatase)
BOEA	ethyl biscoumacetate
bol *bolus*	a large pill
BOMA	bilateral otitis media, acute
BOP	Buffalo orphan prototype (viruses)
bot	botanical, botany
BOW	bag of water (amniotic sac)
BP	Bachelor of Pharmacy
BP	basal state, post-absorptive
BP	bed pan
BP	biparietal (diameter of head)
BP	birth place
BP	blood pressure
BP	buccopulpal
BP	building privilege
↑BP	increasing or elevated blood pressure
↓BP	falling or low blood pressure
bp	bed pan
bp	boiling point
BPB	bromphenol blue (dye)
BPH	benign prostatic hypertrophy
BPL	B-propriolactose
BPLA	blood pressure left arm

BP č̸ P	blood pressure and pulse
BPRA	blood pressure right arm
BR	bathroom
BR	bed rest
BR	boiling range
BR	breathing reserve
Br	bromine
Br	brucella
br	branch
br	breath, breathe
br	brother
br	bruit
brach	brachial
brady	bradycardia
BRB	bright red blood
BR č̄ BRP	bed rest with bathroom privileges
Brit	British
bro	brother
brom	bromide
brn	brown
BRP, BR priv	bathroom privileges
bronch	bronchitis
bronch	bronchogram
bronch	bronchoscope, bronchoscopy
bronch	bronchus

bronchiect	bronchiectasis
BROW	brow presentation (obstetrics)
BRP	bathroom privileges
brph	bronchophony
BRR	breathing reserve ratio
brt	bright
BS	Bachelor of Science
BS	base strap
BS	standard bicarbonate (plasma)
BS	blood sugar
BS	bowel sounds
BS	breath sounds
BS, B/S	broadside (type of impact in accident)
BS	Bureau of Standards
B ∉ S	Bartholin and Skene's glands
bs, @bs	bedside, at bedside
BSA	body surface area
BSA	bovine serum albumin (bovine plasma albumin)
BSA	bowel sounds active
BSB	body surface burn
B Sc	Bachelor of Science
BS ↓ L base	breath sounds diminished left base
BSN	Bachelor of Science in Nursing
BSN	bowel sounds normal
BSO	bilateral salpingo-oophorectomy

BSP	bromsulphalein test
BSS	black silk sutures
BST	blood serologic test
BST	brief stimulus therapy (psychiatry)
BT	bed time
BT	bitemporal (diameter of head)
BT	bitrochanteric (diameter of hips)
BT	bladder tumor
BT	bleeding time
BT	blue tetrazolium
BT	body temperature
BT	bowel tones
BT	brain tumor
BT	breast tumor
BTB	bromthymol blue (dye indicator)
BTR	biceps tendon reflex
BT ¢ R	biceps, triceps and radialis
BTFS	breast tissue (tumor) frozen section
B Th U	British thermal unit
BTPD	body temperature, pressure, dry
BTPS, BTP ¢ S	body temperature, pressure (prevailing atmosphere) and saturation (water vapor)
BTU	British thermal unit
BTW	back to work
Bu	butyl

BU	base of prism up
BU	Bodansky units
Bu	butyl
BUE	both upper extremities
bul	bullet
bull	bulletin
bull *bulliat*	let it boil
BUN	blood urea nitrogen
bun br blk	bundle branch block (heart)
buphth	buphthalmus
BUQ	both upper quadrants
bur	bureau
Burd	Burdick suction
Bur Voc Rehab	Bureau of Vocational Rehabilitation
BUS	Bartholin, urethra and Skene's
but *butryum*	butter
BV *balneum vaporis*	vapor bath
BV	blood volume
BVE	blood volume expander
B vit compl	B vitamin complex
BVL	bilateral vas ligation
BVR	Bureau of Vocational Rehabilitation
BW	bacteriological or biological warfare

BW	bed waiting (list or papers)
BW	birth weight
BW	black and white (milk of magnesia and cascara)
BW	blood wasserman
BW	body weight
BW, bw	twice a week
BWA	bed waiting admission
BX, Bx, bx	biopsy
BX factor	para-amenobenzoic acid
BZD	benzothiadiazine

C	calorie
C	canine
C	capacity (physical)
C	carbohydrate
C	carbon
C	cardiac
C	cast
C	cathode
C	catholic
C	caucasian
C	Celsius
C	centigrade (centigrade temperature is measured on a Celsius scale)
C	centimeter (more often written cm)
C	central
C *centum*	one hundred
C	certified
C	cervical
C	chest
C	chest lead (precordial lead in electrocardiogram)
C *cibus*	food
C *circa*	about, around (usually refers to time)
C	clearance
C	clonus

C   closure

C   coarse

C   coefficient

C   color, colored

C   color sense

C   complement

C   complete

C   complex

C   compound

C   symbol for any constant

C   gallon
  congius

C   contact

C   contingency coefficient

C   contraction

C   control (reference to experiment)

C   cortex

C   Coryne bacterium Example: C diphtheriae

C   rib
  costa

C   costal

C   coulomb (a unit of electricity)

C^1 complement

C#1, C#2 etc.   car number one, car number two etc. in description of an accident

C_1, C_2, C_3, etc.   cervical nerves or vertebrae by number

C-1, C-2, C-3 etc.	cervical nerves or vertebrae by number
C I, C II, C III etc.	cranial nerves
C_1, C_2, C_3, etc.	ribs (costa 1, costa 2, etc.)
C-1, C-2, etc.	sounds below middle C (reaction to tuning fork)
c-1, c-2, c-3, etc.	sounds above middle C (reaction to tuning fork)
C_3 (population)	physically and mentally deficient persons who are products of imperfect development
C_2H_3OH	alcohol
C factor	cleverness factor (psychiatry)
C♀	caucasian female
C♂	caucasian male
c	cast
c	centimeter (usually written cm)
c _centum_	one hundred
c _cibus_	food
c _circa_	about, around (usually refers to time)
c	contact
c _cornu_	horn Example: c inferius = inferior horn of the thyroid cartilage
c	curie
c	current
c̄ _cum_	with
c̄in	within
c̄out	without (usually written s̄)

CA	cancer, carcinoma
CA	cathode
CA	caucasian adult
CA	cervicoaxial
CA	chemical abstracts
CA	chronological age
CA *corpora alata*	cells which perform endocrine function in insects
CA	cortisone acetate
CA	Council Accepted (AMA Council)
CA	cross-sectional area
C/A	caucasian adult
Ca	calcium
Ca	cancer
Ca	cathode
ca	calcium
ca	cancer, carcinoma
ca *circa*	about, around
CAC	cardiac accelerator center
CaCC	cathodal closure clonus
ca cl	calcium chloride
CaCTe	cathodal closure tetanus
CaCx	cancer of cervix
CAD	coronary artery disease
CaDTe	cathodal duration tetanus

CaEdTA	Edathamil calcium disodium
CAF	caucasian adult female
ca gluc	calcium gluconate
CAI	confused artificial insemination
Cal	large calorie (kilogram calorie)
cal	small calorie (gram calorie)
C alb	albumin clearance
calc	calculate
calcd	calculated
calcif	calcification
calef *calefactus*	warm
CAM	caucasian adult male
CAM	chorioallantoic membrane
canc	cancel, cancellation
CaOC	cathodal opening contraction
CaOCl	cathodal opening clonus
CaOTe	cathodal opening tetanus
cap	capacity
cap *capiat*	let him take (pharmacy)
cap	capsule
cap *caput*	head
cap moll *capsula mollis*	soft capsule
caps	capsules

capsul	capsule
caput med *caput medusae*	enlarged veins on skin
CAR	conditioned avoidance response
car	carotid
carb, carbo	carbohydrate
carbon tet	carbon tetrachloride
card	cardiac
card insuff	cardiac insufficiency
cardio	cardiology
cardiol	cardiology, cardiologist
cardio-resp	cardio-respiratory
cart	cartilage
CAS	cerebral arteriosclerosis
CAS	Children's Aid Society
CAS	control adjustment strap
CAT	Child's Apperception Test
CAT	College Ability Test
CAT	computer for average transients
cath	cathartic
cath	catheter, catheterize, catheterization
Cath	Catholic
cathar	cathartic
cauc	caucasian
caut	cautiously

CAVD	A battery of four tests of intelligence: Completion, arithmetic, vocabulary and direction
Ca virus	croup associated virus
CB *Chirugiae Baccalaureus*	Bachelor of Surgery
CB	chest-back
CB	contrast bath
Cb	columbrium
CBC	complete blood count
CBD	closed bladder drainage
CBD	common bile duct
CBF	cerebral blood flow
CBG	cortico-steroid binding globulin; transcortin
CBOC	completion of bed occupancy care
CBR	chemical, bacteriological and radiological
CBS	chronic brain syndrome
CC	caucasian child
CC	cellular compartment
CC	Chief Complaint
CC	coefficient of correlation
CC	color and circulation
CC	Commission Certified
CC	common cold
CC	contrast cystogram
CC	craniocervical
CC	critical condition

CC	current complaint
CC	cylinder cast
C ȼ C	cold and clammy
Cc	concave
cc	cubic centimeter
CCA	chick cell agglutination
CCA	chimpanzee coryza agent
CCAT	conglutinating complement absorption test
CCAU	Chick cell agglutination unit (of Asian vaccine)
CCBV	central circulating blood volume
CCCR	closed chest cardiac resusitation
CCC	cathodal closure contraction
CCCl	cathodal closure clonus
CCD #1	chronic cystic disease grade 1
CCE	clubbing, cyanosis, edema
CCF	cephalin cholesterol flocculation
CCI	chronic coronary insufficiency
CCK	cholecystokinin
CCL	Critical Condition List
C ȼ Cl, c ȼ cl	coitus and climax
CCOT	cervical compression overloading test (Spurling test)
C cr	creatinine clearance
CCS	Casualty Clearance Station
CCS	Crippled Children's Service

ccs, cc's	cubic centimeters
CCT	chocolate coated tablet
C ct	colony count (laboratory)
CCTe	cathodal closing tetanus
CCTM	color, circulation, temperature and movement
CCU	Cardiac Care Unit
CCW	counterclockwise
CD	carbon dioxide (CO_2)
CD	Cardiovascular Disease (Medical specialty, sub-specialty of Internal Medicine)
CD, C-D	cervico-dorsal
CD	childhood disease
CD	civil defense
CD	communicable disease (contagious disease)
CD	constant drainage
CD	convulsive disorder
CD	curative dose
CD_{50}	curative dose for 50% of group
CD *conjugata diagonales*	diagonal conjugate (diameter of pelvic outlet)
Cd	cadmium
Cd	candela
Cd	caudal
Cd	cord
CDAA	chlorodiallylacetamide
CDC	calculated date of confinement

CDC	Communicable Disease Center
CDP	cytidine diphosphate
CDS	cervico-dorsal syndrome Example: CDS c̄ → (L) rad N root distrib = cervico-dorsal syndrome with radiation to left radial nerve root distribution
CE	cardiac enlargement
CE	constant error
C-E	chloroform-ether
C ⊄ E	cough and exercise
Ce	cerium
Ce *celeriter*	quickly
CEC	Council for Exceptional Children
Cel	Celsius (scale on which centigrade temperature is recorded)
cen, cent	center, central
Cent, centi	centigrade
cent	centimeter
ceph floc	cephalin flocculation
ceph chol floc	cephalin cholesterol flocculation
CER	conditioned emotional response
cer	cervical
cereb	cerebral
cert	certificate, certified
cerv	cervical
cerv ser	cervical series (xrays)
CES	central excitatory state

CF	carbolfuchsin
CF	case file
CF	caucasian female
CF	chest and left leg (precordial lead paired with left leg lead in electrocardiogram)
CF	Christmas factor (clotting factor)
CF	citovorum factor
CF	complement fixation
CF	counting fingers (psychiatry)
CF	court files
CF	cystic fibrosis
C/F	caucasian female
C/F	counting fingers (psychiatry)
Cf	californium
cf	confero
C factor	cleverness factor (psychiatry)
CFF	critical fusion (flicker) frequency
cfm, cf/m	cubic feet per minute
CFNS	chills, fever, night sweats
CFT	complement fixation test
CFT	continuous flow tub
CG	center of gravity
CG	choking gas (phosgene)
CG	chorionic gonadotrophin
cg	centigram

CGH	chorionic gonadotrophin
cgm	centigram
CGM	central gray matter (spinal cord)
cgs unit	centimeter gram second (system) unit
CH, C-H	crown-heel (length of fetus or newborn infant)
cH	hydrogen ion concentration
ch	chapter
ch	chest
ch	chief
ch	child
ch	chopped
ch	chronic
Ch B *Chirurgiae Baccalaureous*	Bachelor of Surgery
chap	chapter
char	character, characteristic, characterized
CH D *Chirurgiae Doctor*	Doctor of Surgery
CH D	Doctor of Chemistry
CHD	childhood diseases
CHD	congenital heart disease
CHD	coronary heart disease
ChE	cholinesterase
chem	chemical, chemistry
chems	chemistries (refers to blood chemistries)
CHF	congestive heart failure

chg	change
chg'd	changed
chg's	changes
chlor	chloroform
chl	chloride
ChM *Chirurgiae Magister*	Master of Surgery
CHO, CHo	carbohydrate
chol	cholesterol
cholecyst	cholecystectomy
choles, cholest	cholesterol
chol est	cholesterol esters
cholelith	cholelithiasis
CHO, P, F	carbohydrates, proteins and fats
CHP	Child Psychiatry (subspecialty of Psychiatry)
ch px	chicken pox
Chr	chromobacterium
chr	chronic
c hr	candle hour
Chr bac	chromobacterium
Chr Br Syn, Chr B Synd	chronic brain syndrome
chron	chronic
chron	chronological, chronology
CI	chemotherapeutic index
CI	coefficient of intelligence

CI	color index
cib *cibus*	food
CIBHA	congenital inclusion body hemolytic anemia
CIC	cardiac inhibitor center
CIC	Crisis Intervention Clinic (psychiatric emergency clinic)
CICU	cardiac intensive care unit
CIM	cortically induced movement
C_{IN}, C_{in}	insulin clearance
čin	within
čin NL	within normal limits
cir	circuit
cir	circumference, circumferential
circ	circuit
circ	circular
circ	circulation, circulatory
circ	circumference, circumferential
circ meas	circumferential measurements (orthopedic or neurological examination — measurements of extremities)
circ	circumcision
circ ⊄ sen, circ ⊄ sens	circulation and sensation
CIS	central inhibitory state
cit	citrate
cito disp *cito dispensetur*	dispense quickly

ck	check
ck	cook
ckd	checked
ckd	cooked
ckw	clockwise
CL	center line
CL	chest and left arm (leads in electrocardiogram)
CL	clamp lamp
CL	contact lens
CL	capacity of lung
CL	critical list
Cl	chloride
Cl	chlorine
Cl	clinic, clinical
Cl	Clostridium
cl	centiliter (1/100 liter)
cl	clean
cl	clear, cleared
cl	clinic, clinical
cl	clonus
cl	close, closed
cl	closure
classif	classification, classified
clav	clavicle
cld	closed

cld	colored
clin	clinic, clinical
Clin Path	Clinical Pathologist, Clinical Pathology
Clin Proc	clinical procedure
CLL	chronic lymphocytic leukemia
CLML	Current List of Medical Literature
CLO	cod liver oil
Cl Pal	cleft palate
cl red	closed reduction (of fracture)
Cl T	clotting time
C $\cancel{\mathcal{C}}$ L trx	cervical and lumbar traction
Cl void, cl vd	clean voided (urine specimen)
Clysis, clysis	actually a suffix meaning injection of fluids – the entire word will be indicated by the context. It may be hypodermoclysis, proctoclysis, venoclysis, etc.
CM	caucasian male
CM *Chirurgiae Magister*	Master of Surgery
CM	circular muscle
CM	circumferential measurement (of extremities)
CM	costal margin
CM *cras mane*	tomorrow morning (pharmacy)
C/M	caucasian male
Cm	maximum clearance (usually refers to urea clearance)
Cm	complication

Cm	curium
cm	centimeter
cm	complication
cm *cras mane*	tomorrow morning (pharmacy)
CMA	County Medical Association
CMB	carbolic methyl blue
CMC	carboxymethyl cellulose
CMC	carpometacarpal
CMF	cold mitten friction (physical therapy)
CMP	cystosine monophosphate
CMR	cerebral metabolic rate
CMS	circulation, motion and sensation
cms *cras mane sumendus*	to be taken tomorrow morning (pharmacy)
CMU	complex motor unit
CN	caudate nucleus
CN	circulating nurse (operating room)
CN	chloroacetophenone
CN	cranial nerves
CN II, CN III, etc.	cranial nerves by number
(CN)	cyanogen
cn	canned (diet)
cn *cras nocte*	tomorrow night (Pharmacy)
CNE	chronic nervous exhaustion

CNES	chronic nervous exhaustion state
CNI	chronic nerve irritation
CNS	central nervous system
CNS *cras nocte sumendus*	to be taken tomorrow night (pharmacy)
CN sign	cranial nerve sign (poliomyelitis)
CO	cardiac output
CO	central office
CO	Certified Orthotist
CO	check out
CO	commanding Officer
CO	crossovers (genetics)
C/O, C/o	(under) care of Example: C/o J. Jones, M.D.
C/O	check out
C/O, c/o	complains of
CO_2	carbon dioxide
CO_2 comb	carbon dioxide combining power
Co	cobalt
Co	coenzyme
Co	county
Co_2-O_2	carbogen
Co A	coenzyme A
Co I, II	coenzyme I, coenzyme II etc.
COA	condition on admission
coag	coagulase

coag	coagulate, coagulation
coag time	coagulation time
COC	cathodal opening contraction
coc	coccygeal
coch *cochleare*	spoonful
coch amp *cochleare amplum*	tablespoonful (approximately ½ ounce)
cochl *chochleare*	spoonful
coch mag *cochleare magnum*	tablespoonful (approximately ½ ounce)
coch med *chochleare medium*	desertspoonful (2 fluid drams)
coch mod *cochleare modicum*	desertspoonful (2 fluid drams)
coch parv *cochleare parvum*	teaspoonful (1 fluid dram)
COCl	cathodal opening clonus
coct *coctio*	boiling
Cod	codeine
COD	chemical oxygen demand
coef, coeff	coefficient
COEPS	cortical originating extrapyramidal system
cog	cognate
COH	carbohydrate
Coher	coherent
col	collateral

col   colony (bacteriology)

col   color, colored

col   column

col, colat   strained
  colatus

colen   let them be strained
  colentur

colet   let it be strained
  coleatur

coll   collect, collection

coll   colloidal

coll   eye wash
  collyrium

collat   collateral

collat circ   collateral circulation

Colles fx   fracture of both bones of distal forearm

collun   nose wash (irrigation)
  collunarium

collut   mouth wash
  collutorium

coll vol   collective volume

collyr   eye wash
  collyrium

colost   colostomy

colp   colporrhaphy (vaginal repair)

col/temp   color, temperature

com   comminuted

com   common

com	communicable
comb	combative
comb	combination, combined, combining
comf	comfortable
comm	comminuted
comm	commission
comm	committee
comm	communicable
comm cer *commotio cerebri*	cerebral concussion
commin	comminuted
commun	communicable
commun dis	communicable disease
comp	comparable, comparative, compare
comp	compensate, compensated, compensation
comp	composed of, composition
comp	compound
comp	compress, compressible
Comp case	Workman's Compensation case
compd	compound
compd	compressed
compl	complains, complaint
compl	complete, completed
compl, complic	complicated, complication
compl	complementary

compn	composition
compr	compressed, compression
comprn	compression
compt	competent
con *contra*	against
conc	concentrate, concentration, concentrated
concd	concentrated
concentr	concentrate, concentrated, concentration
concis *conciscus*	cut
concn	concentration
cond	condense, condensed
cond, condn	condition
cond	conductivity, conductor
conduct	conductivity, conductor
cond ref	conditioned reflex
cond milk	condensed milk
cond resp	conditioned response
CONELRAD	control of electromagnetic radiation
conf *confectio*	prescription (pharmacy)
conf	conference
conf	confined
conf, confus	confused
cong	congenital

cong	congested
cong *congius*	gallon
congen	congenital
conj	conjunctiva
conjug	conjugate
cons *conserva*	conserve, keep
cons	consonation
cons	consult, consultation, consultant
conserv	conservative (treatment)
consol	consolidation
consperg *conspergere*	to dust or sprinkle
const	constant
constit	constituency, constituent
constit	constitutional
consult	consultation, consultant
cont	contain, contained, containing
cont	content, contents
cont	continue, continued, continuously
cont *contusus*	contusion, contused (bruised)
contag	contagious, contagion
cont'd	continued
conter *contere*	rub together

contg	containing
contin *continuetur*	let it be continued (pharmacy)
contin	continue, continued, continuing
contr	contract, contracted, contraction
contr	contracture (orthopedic — a permanent muscular contraction due to tonic spasm or to loss of muscular equilibrium)
contra, contra ind	contraindicated, contraindication
contralat *contralateral*	on the opposite side
cont rem *continuantur remedia*	continue medication
cont Rx	continue medication, continue treatment (Rx indicates "that which is ordered")
contus	contusion, bruise
conv	convalescence, convalescent
conv	convergence
conv	convulsion
conv strabis	convergent strabismus
converg	convergence
coop	cooperate, cooperative, cooperation
coor	coordination
coor AMR	coordination and alternate motion rate
COP	colloid osmotic pressure
COPE	chronic obstructive pulmonary emphysema
coq *coque*	boil

coq in s a   boil insufficient water
  coque in sufficiente aqua

coq s a   boil properly
  coque secundum artum

COR   custodian of records

Co R   congo red

cor   correct, corrected, corrective, correction

corr, corresp   correspond, correspondence, ocrresponding

cort   cortex

cort   cortical

cos   cosine

cosec   cosecant

cot, cotan   cotangent

COTe   cathodal opening tetanus

CP   capillary pressure

CP   cerebral palsy

CP   Certified Prosthetist

CP   chemically pure

CP   Child Psychiatrist, Child Psychiatry, Child Psychology

CP   closing pressure (spinal puncture)

CP   constant pressure

CP   right ventricular failure (heart)
  cor pulmonale

CP   creatinine phosphate

CP   cystoscopy and (retrograde) pyelogram

C ȼ P   complete and painfree (range of motion)

cp	compare
cp	candle power
cp	centipoise
CPAH, C_{PAH}	clearance p-aminohippuric acid
CPC	chronic passive congestion
CPC	clinicopathological conference
CPD	cephalopelvic disproportion
cpd	compound
cpds	compounds
CPE	complete physical examination
CPH	Certificate of Public Health
CPI	California Psychological Inventory (test)
CPI	Constitutional Psychopathic Inferior
CPK	creatinine phosphokinase
cpm	counts per minute
cpm	cycles per minute
CPP	cyclopentenophenanthrene
C_3 pop	population of physically or mentally imperfectly developed persons
CPR	cardio-pulmonary resusitation
CPR	centripetal rub (Physical therapy)
CPR	chlorophenyl rub
cps	cycles per second
CPT	combining power test
C &cancel;c P trx	cervical and pelvic traction

CPX, C Px	complete physical examination
CPZ	chloropromazine
CR, C-R	cardiorespiratory
CR	chest and right arm (precordial lead paired with right arm lead in electrocardiogram)
CR	clinical records
CR	closed reduction Example: CR dist rt rad = closed reduction distal right radius
CR	clot retraction
CR	coefficient of fat retention
CR	conditioned reflex
CR	conditioned response
CR	cresyl red
CR	critical ratio
CR, C-R	crown-rump (length of fetus)
Cr	chromium
^{51}Cr	radioactive isotope of chromium
Cr	specific heat at constant volume
Cr	coordination
Cr	creatinine
Cr	crown-rump (length of fetus)
Cr II, etc.	cranial nerves by number
cr *cras*	tomorrow
cr, cran	cranial
crast *crastinus*	for tomorrow

CR ∉ C	closed reduction and cast
CRD	chronic respiratory disease
CRD	complete reaction of degeneration
CRE	chronic rheumatic endocarditis
creat	creatinine
crem, cremas	cremasteric
crep	crepitation, crepitant, crepitus
CRF	corticotrophine releasing (regulating) factor
CRI	chemical rust inhibiting
CRI	Cold Running Intelligibility (test for hearing continuous speech)
crit	hematocrit
crit	critical
CRL	Certified Record Librarian
CRO	cathode ray oscilloscope
CROM	cervical range of motion
CrP	creatine phosphate
CRP	C-reactive protein
CRPA	C-reactive protein antiserum
CRS	Colon and Rectal Surgery
CRT	Cardiac Resusitation Team
CRT	cathode ray tube
CRT	complex reaction time
cr vesp *cras vespere*	tomorrow evening
crys, cryst	crystal, crystalline, crystallized, crystallization

CS	Caesarian Section
CS	central supply
CS	chest strap
CS	chief of staff
CS	concentrated strength (solution)
CS	conditioned stimulus
CS	convalescent status
CS	coronary sinus
CS *corpus stiatus*	striate body
CS	corticosteroid
CS	current strength
CS	Cushing's syndrome
C/S	cycles per second
C/S effect	**cough/sneeze effect**
C ¢ S	calvarium and scalp
C ¢ S	cough and sneeze Example: LBP aggrav by C E = low back pain aggravated by cough and sneeze
C ¢ S	culture and sensitivity
Cs	conscious, consciousness
Cs	standard clearance (urea clearance)
cs	case
cs	conscious, consciousness
CSC	cornea, sclera and conjunctiva (eyes)
CSC *coup sur coup*	small doses at frequent intervals (pharmacy)
csc	cosecant

C sect	Caesarian section
CSF	cerebrospinal fluid
CSF-WR	cerebrospinal fluid, Wasserman reaction
CSM	cerebrospinal meningitis
C sp	cervical spine
CSR	central supply room
CSR	corrected sedimentation rate
CSS	chewing, sucking, swallowing
CST	convulsive shock therapy
CSU	Central Statistical Unit (Venereal Disease Research Laboratory)
CT	cervical traction
CT, C-T	cervical-thoracic area, cervicothoracic area
CT, C-T	cervico thoracic syndrome Example: CT snyd c̆ lt ulnar N rad = cervicothoracic syndrome with left ulnar nerve radiation
CT	circulation time
CT	clear tones (heart)
CT	coated tablet
CT	compressed tablet
CT	connective tissue
CT	continued treatment
CT	total content carbon dioxide
CT	continuous flow tub
CT	corneal transplant
CT	corrective therapy

C ∉ T	color and temperature
C_T 1824	clearance of Evans blue
CTA, CTa	catamenia
CTBM	cetyltrimethylammonium bromide (nerve blocking agent)
CTC	chlortetracycline
C-T-L	cervical, thoracic, lumbar
ctn	cotangent
C ∉ T, N BLE	color and temperature normal, both lower extremities
CTP	cytidine triphosphate
ctr	center
C trx	cervical traction
CTU	centigrade thermal unit
C tx	cervical traction
CT zone	chemoreceptor trigger zone (vomiting area in medulla)
CU	clinical unit
Cu	copper
cu	cubic
cu cm	cubic centimeter
CUD	cause undetermined
cu ft	cubic foot
cu in	cubic inch
cuj	of which, of any
cujus	

cuj lib *cujus libet*	of any you please
cult	culture
cu m	cubic meter
cu mm	cubic millimeter
CUR	cysto-urethro-rectocele
cur	curative
cur	current
curat *curatio*	a dressing
CUS, CU spec	catheterized urine specimen
cu yd	cubic yard
CV	cardiac volume
CV	cardiovascular
CV	cervical vertebra
CV	coefficient of variation
CV	concentrated volume (solution)
CV	conducting veins
CV *conjugata vera*	true conjugate diameter of pelvic outlet
CV	costo-vertebral
CV, cv *cras vespere*	tomorrow evening
Cv	(specific heat at) constant volume
CVA	cardiovascular accident
CVA	cerebrovascular accident
CVA	costovertebral angle

CVAT, CVA T, CVA tend	costovertebral tenderness
CVC, CV cath	central venous catheter
CVD	cardiovascular disease
CVD	cerebrovascular disease
CVI	cardiovascular incident
CV	cardiac volume
CV status	cardiovascular status
C viruses	coxsackie viruses
CVO *conjugata vera obstetrica*	obstetric conjugate diameter (true conjugate oblique)
CVP	central venous pressure
CVR	cardiovascular, respiratory
CVR	cerebrovascular resistance
CW	chemical warfare
CW	continuous wave
CW	crutch walking
CWBTS	capillary whole blood true sugar
CWP	childbirth without pain
cwt	hundred weight
Cx	cervix
Cx, cx	convex
Cx	cervical
Cy	cyanogen
cy, cyan	cyanosis, cyanotic

Cyan DA   diphenylcyanoarsine — a toxic agent proposed for
                              chemical warfare

cyath   glassful
 cyathus

cyath vin   wine glass
 cyathus vinarius

cyc   cyclotron

cyl   cylinder (cast) orthopedics

cyl   cylindrical (lens) ophthalmology

cysto   cystogram, cystoscope, cystoscopy

cytol   cytology

cyt sys   cytochrome system

D	absorbed dose
D	daughter
D	day
D	dead
D	dead space
D	deceased
D (Not an abbreviation)	deci (a prefix meaning 1/10)
D	deciduous (teeth)
D	degree
D	density
D	dermatologist, dermatology (designation of medical specialty)
D	deuterium
D	developed
D	deviation
D *dexter, dextra, dextro*	right
D	dextrorotary
D	dextrose
D	diagnosis
D	diameter
D	diathermy
D	diffusion constant
D	diopter
D (forms)	diphtheroid forms
D	disease

D	distal
D	diverticulum
D	divorced
D	dorsal
D	doubtful
D	duration
D_1 D_2 D_3 etc	dorsal (thoracic) nerves and/or vertebrae by number
2D	second degree erythemal dose
3D	third degree erythemal dose
d *da*	give
d	date
d	daughter
d	day
d	dead, deceased, died Example: F d ca = father died of cancer
d	deadspace
d	degree
d	density
d *dentur*	let them be given (pharmacy)
d *detur*	let it be given (pharmacy)
d *dexter, dextra, dextro*	right
d	dextrorotary
d	diameter

d	dorsal
d	dose
d	ductus
d	dyne
1/d	once a day
2/d	twice a day
17 d	modified yellow fever virus
DA	delayed action
DA	disability assistance
DA	District Attorney
D/A	date of accident
D/A	date of admission
Da, da	daughter
Da	diphenularsine chloride, dipehnylchorarsine (Adamsite)
da	day
da (Not an abbreviation)	deca (a prefix meaning 10)
DAH	disordered action of the heart
dal	decaliter
DAM	diacetylmonoxine
DAP	dihydroxyacetone phosphate
DAP (test)	Draw a Person test (psychology)
DAS	dead air space
DAT	diet as tolerated
DAT	Differential Aptitude Test

DAT	diphtheria antitoxin
dau	daughter
DB, D/B	date of birth
DB	diameter of Baudelocque (external conjugate diameter of the pelvis)
DB	distobuccal
Db, db	decibel (unit of measuring loudness)
DBA	dibenzanthracene
DBI–TD	Phenformin hydrochloride
dbl	double
DBP	dibutylphthalate
DBP	distobuccopulpal (planes of teeth)
DBS	depreciated bovine serum
DBS	Division of Biological Standards
DC, D/C	damp, cold (weather)
DC	Dental Corps
DC	Diagnostic Center
DC	dilitation and curettage
DC	diphenulcyanoarsine
DC	direct current (electricity)
DC	discharge, discharged (dismiss)
DC, dc	discontinue, discontinued
DC	Doctor of Chiropractic (chiropractor)
D&C	dilitation and curettage
DCA	desoxycorticosterone acetate

DCc	double concave
Dc'd, dc'd	discontinued
DCF	direct centrifugal flotation
DCG	desoxycorticosterone glucoside
DCH	Diploma of Child Health
DCP	dicalcium phosphate
DCR	direct cortical response
DCx	double convex
DD	dependent drainage
DD	differential diagnosis
DD	discharge by death
DD	discharge diagnosis (final diagnosis)
DD	dry dressing
DD	dying declaration
D→D	discharge to duty
DDA	acetic derivation of DDT (excreted in urine)
dd in d *de die in diem*	from day to day
DDE	derivative of DDT stored in fat
DDS	diaminodiphenyl sulfone
DDS	disability determination service
DDS	Doctor of Dental Surgery
DDsc	Doctor of Dental Science
DDT	dichlorodiphenyl trichoroethane
D/DW, D 5 DW, D 5%Dw	dextrose in distilled water

DE	dose equivalent
D∉E	diet and elimination
DEAE	diethylaminoethanol
DEB	diethylbutanediol
debil	debilitation, debility
deb spis *debita spissitudo*	of proper consistency
dec *decanta*	pour off (pharmacy)
dec	deceased
dec	decimeter
dec	decomposed
dec'd	deceased
dec'd	decomposed
decim	decimeter
decoct	decoction
decomp	decompensate, decompensated
decomp	decompose, decomposed
decompn	decompensation
decompn	decomposition
decr	decrease, decreased
decub	decubitus
de d in d *de die in diem*	from day to day
def	defecate, defecation
def	deferred

def	deficiency, deficient
def	deficit
def	definite
D-FECT	dense fibroelastic connective tissue
defic	deficiency, deficient
deform	deformity
deg	degeneration
deg	degree, degrees
degen	degeneration, degenerative
deglut *degluriatur*	deglutition (swallowing)
d in dup *detur in duplo*	give twice as much
dehyd	dehydrated, dehydration
del	deliver, delivery
del	delusion
deliq	deliquescent
Dem	demerol
dem	demonstrate, demonstrated
Demen Prae	Dementia Praecox
demin	demineralization
dens	teeth
dent	dental, dentist, dentistry, dentition
dent	dentate (toothed, cogged, notched)
dent *dentur*	let them be given

dent tal dos   give of such doses
  dentur tales doses

DEP   diethylpropanediol

dep   deposit

dep   purify
  depuratus

depr   depressed, depression

dept   department

DeR   reaction of degeneration

der, deriv   derivative, derive, derived

derm   dermatologist, dermatology

derm   dermatome

desat   desaturated, desaturation

desc   descendent, descending

descr   describe

desq   desquamation

dest   distill, distilled
  destilla

det   let it be given (pharmacy)
  detur

det in dup   let twice as much be given
  detur in duplo

det in 2 plo   let twice as much be given

detn   determination

dets   let it be given and labeled
  deturet signatur

d et s   give and label
  da et signa

det time	detention time (time doctor detained in Emergency Room, etc.)
detox	detoxification Example: detoxification period — the period of time during which drugs are being withdrawn from an addict
D Ety	disease etiology
dev	develop, developed, development
dev	deviated, deviation
devd	developed
devel	develop, developed, development
dex, dext	dexterity
dex, dext *dexter, dextra, dextro*	right
DF, df	dorsiflexion
DF	dry gas fractional concentration
df	degrees of freedom
DFO	desferrioxamine
D forms	diphtheroid forms
D forms	dwarf forms
DG, dg	diagnose, diagnosis, diagnostic
dg	decigram
dge	drainage
dgtr	daughter
DH	daily habits
DHE 45	dihydroergotomine
DHEW	Department of Health Education and Welfare
DHF	dorsi-hyperflexion

DHO   deuterium hydrogen oxide

DHT   dihydrotachysterol

DI, D/I   date of injury

DI   deterioration index

DI   diabetes insipidus

Di   didymium

dia   diameter

dia   diathermy

diab   diabetes, diabetic

diag   diagonal

diag   diagnosis

diag   diagram

dia lw   long wave diathermy

dia sw   short wave diathermy

diam   diameter

diaph   diaphragm

diaph   diaphysial, diaphysis

diath   diathermy

DIB   Disability Insurance Benefits

dict   dictate, dictated

dieb alt   alternate days
  diebus alternis

dieb secund   every second day
  diebus secundis

dieb tert   every third day
  diebus tertius

diff	difference
diff	differential
Diff, diff	differential white blood cell count
diff diag	differential diagnosis
diff	difficult
DIFP	diisopropylfluorophosphate
Dig, dig	digitalis
dig	digest, digestion
DIH	Diploma of Industrial Health
DIL	daughter in law
dil	dilate, dilated, dilatation
dil	dilute, diluted, dilution
dilat	dilate, dilated, dilatation
diln	dilution
diluc *diluculo*	at daybreak
dilut	dilute, dilution, diluted
dim *dimidius*	make up one half the order (pharmacy)
dim	diminished
dim T	diminished time
dim T	diminished tone
dimin	diminished, diminution
d in p aeq *divides in partes aequales*	divide into equal parts (pharmacy)
DIP	desquamative interstitial pneumonia

DIP	distal interphalangeal
Dip	diphtheria
Dip Amer Bd P N	Diplomate of the American Board of Psychiatry and Neurology
diph	diphtheria
diop	diopter
DIR	disturbed interpersonal relationships
Dir	Director
dir	directory
dir prop *directione propria*	with proper directions
Dis, dis	disabled, disability
dis	discomfort
dis	disease
dis	distance
dis	distribution
disab	disability, disabled
disart, disartic	disarticulation
disc	discharge
disc	discomfort
disch, dischg	discharge
disch AMA	discharged against medical advice
Disch PHC	discharged to post-hospital care
discom, discomf	discomfort
disl, disloc	dislocate, dislocated, dislocation
dism	dismiss, dismissed

disord	disorder
disp	dispense, dispensary
disp	disposition
displ	displace, displacement
dissd	dissolved
dissem	disseminate, dissemination, disseminated
dissoc	dissociate, dissociation
dist	distal
dist	distance
dist	distended
dist	distilled
dist	distinguish, distinguished
dist f	distinguished from
dist H_2O	distilled water
distr	distressed
distr, distrib	distribute, distributed, distribution
DIT	diiodotyrosine
div	divide, division
div	divorced
div in P aeq *divides in partes aequales*	divide into equal parts
DJD	degenerative joint disease
dk	dark Example: dk brn = dark brown
DK	diet kitchen
DKA	Didn't keep appointment

dkg   decagram

dkl   decaliter

dkm   dekameter

DL   Danger List (Critical List)

DL   difference limen (threshold)

D/L   date of liability, date of loss (insurance)

D-L   Donath-Landsteiner (antibody)

dl   decaliter

DL ¢ B   direct laryngoscopy and bronchoscopy

DLE   disseminated lupus erythematosis

DM   dermatologist, dermatology

DM   diabetes mellitus

DM   diastolic murmur

DM   diphenylamine chlorarsine (Adamsite)

DM   Doctor of Medicine

dm   decimeter

DMD   Doctor of Dental Medicine
 Dentariae Medicinae Doctor

DME   Director of Medical Education

DMF   decayed, missing, and filled (teeth)

DMS   dermatomyositis

DMS   Director of Medical Service

DMS   Doctor of Medical Science

DN   dicrotic notch

Dn, dn   decinem

DNA	deoxyribonucleic acid
DNA	does not apply
DNB	dinitrobenzene
DNE	Director of Nursing Education
DNKA	did not keep appointment
DNR	dorsal nerve root
D/NR, D:N ratio	dextrose to nitrogen ratio in urine
DNS	did not show (for appointment)
D/NS	dextrose in normal saline
D5NS, D5%/NS	5% dextrose in normal saline
DO	diamine oxidase
DO	Doctor of Optometry
DO	Doctor of Osteopathy
do	ditto
DOA	date of admission
DOA	dead on arrival
DOB	date of birth
DOB	Doctor's Order Book
DOC	deoxycorticosterone
doc	document, documentation
DOCA	deoxycorticosterone acetate (drug for Addison's disease)
DOCF	deoxycorticosterone flucoside
DOE	deoxyephedrine hyrochloride
DOE	dyspnea on exertion (exertional dyspnea)

DOI   date of injury

dol   pain
  dolor

dom   domestic

don   until
  donec

don alv sol fuerit   until bowel is open
  donec alvus solula fuerit

D Oph   Doctor of Ophthalmology

dor   dorsal

dorm   dormant

dorna   desoxyribonucleic acid (DNA)

dorsi, dorsifl   dorsiflexion

DOS   day of surgery

dos   dosage

dos   doses

DOSS   distal over shoulder strap

DOT   date of transfer

DOT   Dictionary of Occuptational Titles

DOT   Diploma of Occupational Therapy

doz   dozen

DP   deep pulse

DP   degree of polymerization

DP   dementia praecox

DP   diphosgene

DP   proper directions
  directiones propria

DP	displaced person
DP	Doctor of Pharmacy
DP	dorsalis pedis
DP	dyspnea (computer compatible)
DPA	diphenyl amine
DPD	Department of Public Dispensary
DPDA	phosphorodiamidic anhydride
DPH	Department of Public Health
DPH	Diploma in Public Health
DPH	Doctor of Public Health
DPI	diphtheria and pertussis immunization
DPM	Diploma in Psychologic Medicine
DPN	diphosphopyridine nucleotide
DPNase	enzyme hydrolizing DPN
DPT	diphtheria-pertussis-tetanus immunization
DQ	deterioration quotient
dr	drain
dr	dram
dr	dressing
Dr.	doctor
DR	reaction of degeneration (muscle fibers)
DR	Diagnostic Radiology
DR	dining room
DR	dorsal root
dr ap	dram apothecary weight

DRC$_1$ DRC$_2$ etc.	dorsal root cervical
DRD	dorsal root dilator
D reg	diseased region
drg	drainage, draining
DRL #2, DRL #3 or DRL$_1$, DRL$_2$	dorsal root lumbar by number
DRNA	desoxyribose nucleic acid
drng	drainage, draining
DRP	Deutsches-Reichs Patent
D Rnt	diagnostic roentgenology
DRQ	discomfort relief quotient
DRR	dorsal root reflex
DRS$_1$, DRS$_2$, etc	dorsal root sacral by number
drsg	dressing
DRT$_1$, DRT$_2$, etc	dorsal root thoracic by number
DS	dead air space
DS	deep sedative
DS	dilute strength (solution)
DS	dioptric strength (lens)
DS	Doctor of Science
D/s	dextrose in saline
DSC	Doctor of Surgical Chiropody (chiropodist)
D Sc	Doctor of Science
DSCT	dorsal spinocerebellar tracts
DSD	discharge summary dictated

DSD	dry sterile dressing
DSF	dry sterile fluff
DSG	dry sterile gauze
DSP	decreased sensory perception
DST	daylight saving time
DT, DTs	delirium tremens
DT	distance test
DT	dorsalis tibialis
DT	duration of tetany
D/T	date of treatment
D/T, dt	due to
D c̄ T	date and time
DTD, dtd *datur tales dosis*	give (number) such doses
DTN	diphtheria toxin normal
DTP	diphtheria-tetanus-pertussis (immunization)
DTP	digital tingling on pressure
DTP	diphtheria, tetanus, pertussis
DTP	distal tingling on percussion
dtr	daughter
DTR	deep tendon reflexes
DTR/NL	deep tendon reflexes within normal limits
DTR = c̄ act	deep tendon reflexes equal and active
DT's, Dt's, dt's	delirium tremens
DTUS, d tx US	diathermy, traction and ultra sound

DTV   due to void (patient should void by this time)

DU   diagnosis undertermined

DU   dog unit

DU   duodenal ulcer

DUB   dysfunctional uterine bleeding

duod   duodenal, duodenum

dup   duplicate, duplication

dur   duration, during
  durante

dur dol   duration of pain, while pain lasts
  durante dolore

DV   dependent variable

DV   dilute volume

D $\notni$ V   discs and vessels (eyes)

dv   double vibrations

DVA   Department of Veteran's Affairs

DVA   duration of voluntary apnea (test)

dvlp   develop, development

DVR   Department of Vocational Rehabilitation

DW, D/W   dextrose and water (often the first nourishment
                                       offered newborn infants)

D5W, D5%/W   5% dextrose in water

DW   distilled water

DW   doing well

DW, impr   doing well, improving

dwt   pennyweight
  denarius weight

Dx, dx	diagnosis
Dx, dx	disease
dx	difficulties
↑dx or ↗dx	increased difficulties
Dy	dysprosium
dyn	dynamics
dysp	dyspnea, dyspneic
dz	dozen

E	each
E	early
E	edema
E	einsteinium
E	electrical affinity
E	electromotive force
E	emmetropia
E	enema
E	energy
E	enzyme
E	Escherichia
E	examiner
E	experiment, experimenter
E	expired
E	extension
E	eye
e	early
e	electric charge
e	electron
e	erg
$\mathcal{E}$ *et*	and
E 50%N	extension 50% of normal
E substance	excitor substance
E voltage	electrical voltage

E 107	tribromoethanol (Avertin)
EA	educational age
ea	each
EAC	external auditory canal
ead *eadem*	the same
EAE	experimental allergic encephalomyelitis
EAHF	eczema, allergy, hay fever
EAP	Emergency Aid Program
EA-TDA	2 acetylamino-1,3,4-thiadiazole
E ∉ H	environment and heredity
E ∉ M	endocrine and metabolic
Ea-R	Entartungs-Reaktion (reaction of degeneration)
EB	east bound (in description of auto accident)
EB	elbow bearing
Eb	erbium
EBL	estimated blood loss
EBL/S	estimated blood loss/surgery
EBS	elastic back strap
EC	enteric coated
EC	entering complaint
EC	ether and chloroform
EC	expiratory center
EC	external conjugate (pelvic measurement)
ECB	electric cabinet bath

ECCE	extracapsular cataract extraction
E-C coupling	excitation-contraction coupling
ECF	extended care facility (convalescent home)
ECF	extra cellular fluid
ECG	electrocardiogram
echo	echoencephalogram
echo syst	echo systole (heart sound)
ECHO virus	enterocytopathogenic human orphan virus
eclamp	eclampsia
eclec	eclectic
EC mix	ether chloroform mixture
E coli	Escherichia coli
ECP	free cytoporphyrin in erythrocytes
ECPR	external cardiopulmonary resusitation
ECT	electroconvulsive therapy (psychiatry)
ect	ectopic
etc *et cetera*	and so forth
ED	effective dose
ED	elbow disarticulation
ED	entering diagnosis
ED	erythema dose
ED	ethyl dichlorarsine
ED	exertional dyspnea
ED_{50}	median effective dose (effective for 50% of group)

Ed	editor
ed	edema
ed	edition
EDC	estimated date of confinement, expected date of confinement (obstetrics)
EDC	expected delivery, Caesarian
EDD	estimated due date (obstetrics)
edem turb	edematous turbinates
EDN	electrodesiccation
EDR	effective direct radiation
EDR	electrodermal response
EDTA	ethylenediaminetetracetic acid (Edathamil)
educ	education, educational
E DX	electrodiagnosis
EE, E ¢ E	eyes and ears
EECG	electroencephalogram
EEE	eastern equine encephalitis
EEG	electroencephalogram
EENT	eyes, ears, nose and throat
EF	equivalent focus
EF	essential findings
EFA	essential fatty acids
eff	effect, effective, effects
eff	efferent
eff	efficient

eff	effusion
EFP	effective filtration pressure
EFR	effective filtration rate
e g *exempli gratii*	for example
EGG	electrogastrography
E ¢ H	environment and heredity (psychiatry)
eH	oxidation reduction potential
EHBF	extra hepatic blood flow
EHF	exophthalmos-hyperthyroid factor
EHF	extremely high frequency
EHL	effective half life (radioactive substance)
EHL	extensor hallucis longus
EHPT	Eddy hot plate test
EJ	elbow jerk
ejusd *ejusdem*	of the same
EK, EKG	electrocardiogram (from German spelling)
EKY	electrokymogram
EL	elopement status
el	elbow
ELB	elbow lock billet
elb	elbow
elect	elective
elect	electric
elect	electuary

elect surg	elective surgery
elev	elevate, elevation, elevator
elix	elixir
EM	electron microscope
EM	emmetropia (normal vision)
EM	erythema multiform
EM	excreted mass
E-M	Embden-Meyerhoff (glycolytic pathway)
E ⊄ M	endocrine and metabolic
em	emmetropia (normal vision)
e/m	ratio of charge to mass
EMB	eosin methylene blue
emb	embolus
emb	embryo
embry	embryology
EMC virus	encephalomyocarditis virus
emer, emerg	emergency
EMF	electromotive force
EMF	erythrocyte maturing factor
EMG	electromyogram, electromyography
EMIC	emergency mother and infant care
emot	emotion, emotional
EMP	electromagnetic pulse
emp _emplastrum_	plaster

emp	employee, employer, employment
e m p *ex modo prescripto*	in the manner prescribed, as ordered
Emp	emperin
Emp comp	emperin compound
emph, emphys	emphysema
empl	employee, employer, employment
EMS	electrical muscle stimulation
EMU, emu	electromagnetic unit
emul, emuls	emulsion
EN	electronarcosis (Psychiatry)
en	enema
endo, endocr	endocrine, endocrinology
endos, endost	endosteal
endo-trach	endo-tracheal
enem	enema
enl	enlarge, enlarged, enlargement
ENT	ears, nose and throat
entom	entomology
EOA	examination, opinion and advice
EOG	electrooculography
EOM	extra ocular movements
EOM	extra ocular muscles
EOM F &c Conj	extra ocular movements full and conjugate
EOM	external otitis media

E of M	error of measurement
EOP	Emergency Out Patient
eos, eosins	eosinophils
EP	edible portion
EP	protoporphyrin (free in erythrocytes)
ep	epithelial, epithelium
EPA	exact posteroanterior (position)
ep cells	epithelial cells
EPH	extensor proprius hallucis
ephed	ephedrine
epi	epinephrine
epigast	epigastrium
epil	epilepsy, epileptic
epineph	epinephrine
epiph	epiphysis
epis	episiotomy
epis	episode, episodes, episodic
epis	epistaxis
epistom *epistomium*	a stopper
epith	epithelial, epithelium
epp	end plate potential
EPR	electrophrenic respiration
EPS	exophthalmus-producing substance
ep's	epithelial cells

EPSP	excitatory postsynaptic potential
EPTS	existed prior to service (civil, industrial or military)
EQ	education quotient
eq	equal, equivalent
eqpt, equip	equipment
equiv	equivalent
equiv	equivocal
ER	Emergency Room
ER	endoplasmic reticulum
ER	equivalent roentgen
ER	expiratory reserve
ER	extended release
ER	external resistance
ER	external rotation
E ₵ R	equal and reactive (reflexes – usually pupils)
E ₵ R	examination and report
ERD	evoked response detector
ERG	electroretinogram
ERPF	effective renal plasma flow
eruct	eructation
ERV	expiratory reserve volume
Ery	erysipelothrix
eryth	erythema
eryth	erythrocytes (red blood cells)

ES	elastic suspensor
ES	electrical stimulation
ES	Emergency Service
ES	estimated normal value, (standard)
ES	extra systole
Esch	Escherichia
ESF	erythropoietic stimulating factor
esoph	esophageal, esophagoscopy, esophagus
ESP	extra sensory perception
esp, espec	especially
ESR	electron spin resonance
ESR	erythrocyte sedimentation rate
ess	essence
ess	essentially
EST	electroshock therapy
est	estimate, estimated
esth	esthetic
est wt, est wgt	estimated weight
ESU	electrostatic unit
E substance	excitor substance
ET	educational therapy
ET	esotropia
et (Not an abbreviation)	latin word for and
et	ethyl
et	etiology

ETAB	extra thoracic assisted breathing (Cuirass-type respirator with positive and negative phases)
et al *et alibi*	and elsewhere
et al *et alii*	and others
etc *et cetera*	and so forth
ETF	electron-transferring flavoprotein
eth	ether
eths	ethmoids
etiam (Not an abbreviation)	also, besides
etiol	etiology
ETOH	ethyl alcohol
etiol undet	etiology undetermined
etiol unk	etiology unknown
ETKM, ETKTM	every test known to man
et seq *et sequens*	and the following
et seq *et sequentes*	and those that follow
ETT	endotracheal tube
Eu	european
Eu	europium
eust	eustachian
eutroph	eutrophia, eutrophic
EV	extra vascular (interstitial fluid)
ev	electron volt

ev	eversion
evac	evacuate
eval	evaluate, evaluation
evap	evaporate, evaporation
evapn	evaporation
ever	eversion
evid	evidence, evident, evidenced by
EW	Emergency Ward
ex (Not an abbreviation)	a latin word meaning from, out of
ex	exacerbate, exacerbated, exacerbation
ex	exaggerate, exaggerated
ex	examine, examiner, examination
ex	exercise
exac	exacerbate, exacerbated, exacerbation
exag	exaggerate, exaggerated, exaggeration
exam	examine, examination, examiner
exc	excel, excellent
exc	except
exc	excision
excr	excrete, excreted, excretion
exch	exchange
excis	excise, excision
exec	executive
exer	exercise

ex gr *ex grupa*	from the group
exh	exhibit, exhibition
exhib *exhibeatur*	let it be given (pharmacy)
exhib	exhibit, exhibition
exog	exogenous
exoph	exophthalmia
exos	exostosis
exp	expansion
exp	expect, expected, expecting
exp	experience
exp	experiment, experimental
exp	expire, expiration (cessation of life)
exp	expiration (respiration)
exp	expose
exper	experience
exper	experiment, experimental
expir	expiration, expiratory
expl	explain
expl	explore, exploratory, exploration
exp = sat	expansion equal and satisfactory (chest)
expt	expect
expt	expectorate
exptl	experimental
ext	extend, spread

ext	extend, extension
ext	extensive
ext	extensor
ext	exterior
ext	external
ext	externe
ext	extract Example: fl ext = fluid extract
ext	extracted, extraction Example: tooth extraction
ext	extreme
ext	extremity
extd	extended
extd	extracted
extens	extension
extens	extensor
ext aud	external auditory (canal)
extentab	extended action tablet
ext fl	fluid extract
extrav	extravasation
extrem	extremity
ext rot	external rotation
↑ ext rot	increased external rotation (usually indicating increase beyond normal limits)
↓ ext rot	decreased external rotation
extub	extubate, extubated, extubation
exud	exudate, exuded

F *Fahrenheit*	Fahrenheit
F	fair
F	farad
F	father
F	Fellow (belonging to a fellowship or society)
F	French (catheter size)
F	fundus
f	father
f	farad
f	female
f *facer*	to make
f *fiant*	let them be made
f *fiat*	let it be made
f	fibrous
f	field (vision)
f	finger breadth (gross measurement of position of fundus, neck flexion range, enlargement of liver, etc)
f	five
f	flexion
f	fluid
f	focal
f	following
f	foot

f	form
f	formula, formulary
f	fraction, fractional
f	fracture
f	french (indication of catheter size)
f	frequency
f	from
f	frontal
f	full
f	general function
f	fundus
f (followed by number)	focal length
F_1, F_2, f_1, f_2, etc.	first filial generation, second filial generation, etc.
f	freon
FA	fatty acid
FA	femoral artery
FA	filterable agent
FA	First Aid
FA	folic acid
FA	forearm
FA	fortified aqueous (solution)
f℥	fluid ounce
f℈	fluid dram
FA	functional activities
FAA sol	formalin, acetic, alcohol solution

FAB	functional arm brace
Fabere	flexion, abduction, external rotation and extension
fac *facere*	to make
FACD	Fellow American College of Dentists
FACHA	Fellow American College of Hospital Administrators
facil	facilitate, facilitation, facilitory
FACP	Fellow American College of Physicians
FACS	Fellow American College of Surgeons
FACT	Flanagan Aptitude Classification Test
FAD	flavin adenine dinucleotide
$FADH_2$	flavin adenine dinucleotide, reduced form
Fadire	flexion, adduction, internal rotation and extension (reverse of Fabere)
Fahr	Fahrenheit
fam	family
FAMA	Fellow American Medical Association
fam doc	family doctor
fam hist	family history
fam per par	familial periodic paralysis
fam phys	family physician
FANSS & M	fundus anterior, normal size and shape, and mobile
FAP	fatty acids polyunsaturated
FAPA	Fellow American Psychiatric Association

FAPHA	Fellow American Public Health Association
FAR	Flight Aptitude Rating
far	farad, faradic
fasc, fasci	fasciculation
FB	finger breadth
FB	foreign body
FBCOD	foreign body cornea, right eye
FBCOS	foreign body cornea, left eye
FBR	Frischblut reaction (syphilis)
FBS	fasting blood sugar
fc	foot candles
FCA	fracture, complete, angulated
FCAP	Fellow American College of Pathologists
FCC	fracture, complete, compound
FCCC	fracture, complete, compound, comminuted
FCD	fracture, complete, deviated (usually refers to nasal fracture)
fcly	facelying
FCP	final common pathway (neurology)
fct	function
FCVD	fracture, complete, varus deformity
FD	family doctor
FD	fan douche
FD	fatal dose
FD	focal distance

FD_{50}	fatal dose for 50% of subjects
Fd	fundus
fd	frequency times deviation
FDA	fronto-dextro-anterior (fetal position)
FDA	Food and Drug Administration
FDDC	ferric dimethyl dithiocarbonate
fdg	feeding
FDLMP	first day of last menstrual period
FDP	fronto-dextro-posterior (fetal position)
FDT	fronto-dextro-transverse (fetal position)
5 FDU	5 flurodeoxyuridine
FE	forced expiratory
Fe *ferrum*	iron
fe	female
feb *febre*	fever
feb dur *febre durante*	while fever continues
FECT	fibroelastic connective tissue
Fel	Fellow (of Academy, etc.)
fem	female, feminine
fem	femoral, femur
fem intern *femoribus internus*	inner thighs
FER	flexion, extension and rotation
fert'd	fertilized

ferv	boiling
fervens	
Fe SO$_4$	ferrous sulfate (iron sulfate)
fest	festination
fet	fetus
FEV	forced expiratory volume
FF	fat free (diet)
FF	filtration faction
FF	fixing fluid
FF	force fluids
FF	forward flexion
FF	foster father
ff	forward flexion
ff	the following
f → f	finger to finger
f → f & f → n	finger to finger and finger to nose (neurological test)
FFA	free fatty acid
FFC	free from chlorine
FFCS	forearm flexion control strap
FFD	focus to film distance
FFROM	full, free, range of motion
FFFT	forward flexion finger tips to _____ (distance from floor or distance down legs e.g. to knee etc.
FFT	flicker fusion threshold
FH	Family History

FH	fetal heart
FH	Frankfort horizontal (plane of skull)
fh *fiat haustus*	make a draught (pharmacy)
FHR	fetal heart rate
FHS	fetal heart sounds
FHT	fetal heart tones
FI	forced inspiratory
FI	functional inquiry
fib	fiber, fibrous
fib	fibrillation
fib	fibula
fibr, fibrill	fibrillation
FICS	Fellow International College of Surgeons
fig	figure
FIGLU	forminino-L-glutamic acid
Fig 4	description of Fabere test
FIL	father in law
fil	filament, filamentous
fil	filial
filt	filter, filtered
FIN	fine intestinal needle
F insulin	fibrous insulin
Fior c̄ Cod	Fiorinal with Codeine
Fish conc	Fishberg concentration

Fish dil	Fishberg dilution
Fiss, fiss	fissure
fist	fistula
FJRM	full joint range of motion
FL	filtered load
FL	focal length
Fl	fluorescein (test for eye ulcer)
fl	flank
fl	fluid
fl	flexion
fl	flutter
FLA	fronto-laeva anterior (fetal position)
fla *fiet lege artis*	do according to rule
flac	flaccid
flav *flavus*	yellow
fld	fluid
fl dr	fluid dram
fl drs	fluff dressing
fld ext, fldxt	fluid extract
flex	flex, flexed, flexion, flexor
flex-ext inj	flexion-extension injury
fl ext	fluid extract
flocc	flocculation
fl oz	fluid ounce

FLP	fronto-laeva posterior (fetal position)
FLS	fibrous long spacing
FLT	fronto-laeva transverse (fetal position)
fluor, fluores	fluorescent
fluor	fluoroscopy
flx	flexion
F+ly	fair plus lying
FM	filtered mass
FM	frequency modulation
FM	flavin mononucleotide
FM	foster mother
F-M	Fletcher Motis
FM (x-ray)	full mouth dental x-rays
fm *fiat mistura*	make a mixture
fm	from
FMD	family doctor
FMF	Familial Mediteranean Fever
FMG	fine mesh gauze (used in plastic surgery)
FMH	Family Medical History
FMN	flavin mononucleotide
F-N, F→N	finger to nose (coordination test)
fo	fomentation
FOB	foot of bed
↗FOB	elevate foot of bed

FOOB	feet out of bed (dangle)
fol	follow
fol *folium*	leaf
FOP	Forensic Pathology (subspecialty of Pathology)
for	foreign
for body	foreign body
form	formation, forming
fort *fortis*	strong
FP	Family Physician
FP	final pressure (lumbar puncture)
FP	flat plate (anteroposterior x-ray of abdomen)
FP	flavin phosphate
FP	foot pound
FP	forearm pronated
fp *fiat potio*	make a potion
fp	flexor pollicis longus
fp	foot pound
f pil *fiant pilulas*	make pills (Example: f pil XX = make twenty pills)
FPL	flexor pollicus longus
FPM	filter paper microscopic test
FPM	full passive movements
fpm	feet per minute
fps	feet per second

fps	foot pound second
fps	frames per second
FR	flocculation reaction
FR	frequency of respiration (respiratory rate)
FR	full range
FR	functional residual capacity
F ⊄ R	force and rhythm (pulse)
Fr	francium
frac	fracture
fract	fraction
fract	fracture
fract dos *fracta dosi*	divided doses (pharmacy)
frag	fragile, fragility
frag	fragment, fragmented
frag test	fragility test
FRC	functional residual capacity
frem	fremitus
frem voc *fremitus vocalis*	vocal fremitus
freq	frequency, frequent
frict	friction
Fried test	Friedman test (for pregnancy)
FRJM	full range joint motion
FROM	full range of motion
FR r, Fr r, fr r	friction rub

FS	factor of safety
FS	forearm supinated
FS	forequarter (shoulder)
FS	fracture site
FS	frozen section
F $\cancel{c}$ S	full and soft
F sheet	field sheet
fsa *fiat secundum artem*	do it skillfully
FSB	Family Service Bureau
FSC	fracture, simple, complete
FSCC	fracture, simple, complete, comminuted
FSD	focus to skin distance
FSD	fracture, simple, depressed (skull)
FSH	follicle stimulating hormone
FSS	front support strap
FT	finger tip
ft *fiant*	let them be made (pharmacy)
ft *fiat*	let it be made (pharmacy)
ft	feet, foot
FTA	fluorescein treponema antibody (test)
ft c	foot candle
ft catapl *fiat cataplasma*	let a poultice be made (pharmacy)

ft cerat   let a cerate be made (pharmacy)
  fiat ceratum

ft chart   make powders (pharmacy)
  fiant chartulae

ft collyr   make an eye wash
  fiat collyrium

FTE   full time equivalent

ft emuls   make an emulsion (pharmacy)
  fiat emulsio

ft enem   make an enema
  fiat enema

FTF   finger to finger

ft garg   make a gargle
  fiat gargarisma

ft infus   make an infusion
  fiat infusum

ft injec   make an injection
  fiat injectio

FTKA   failed to keep appointment

ftL   foot Lambert

ft linim   make a liniment
  fiat linimentum

ft mas   let a mass be made (from which powders or pills
  fiat massa   will be made)

ft mas div in pil   make a mass and divide into pills
  fiat massa dividio in pilulae

ft mist   let a mixture be made
  fiat mistura

FTN   finger to nose (coordination test)

FTND   full term, normal delivery

FTNSD   full term, normal, spontaneous delivery

ft sol *fiat solutio*	make a solution
ft suppos *fiat suppositorium*	make suppositories
FTS	fingertips
FTT	finger tips to (indication of range of forward flexion in back examination)
ft ung *fiat unguentum*	make an ointment
FU	follow up
FU (care)	follow up care (post operative or post injury)
5 FU	5 fluorouracil
F u	Finsen unit
FUBAR	fouled up beyond all recognition
funt	function, functional
FUO	fever of undetermined origin
FUOV	follow up office visit (usually written: 1st FUOV etc.)
fus	fusion
fw	fresh water
FWB	full weight bearing (orthopedic)
fx	fracture
fx	friction
FY	fiscal year

G	conductance
G	gingival
G	globular
G	glucose
G	gonidial (bacteriology)
G	gravity
G	unit of force of acceleration due to gravity
G	gravity constant
G	good
G	gram
G	gravida
G	dichlorophen
G_{11}	hexachlorophene
g	conductance
g	gingival
GA	gastric analysis
GA	general anesthesia
GA	general appearance (physical examination)
GA, G/A	gingivoaxial (tooth planes)
G/A quotient	globulin-albumin quotient
Ga	gallium
GABA	gamma aminobutyric acid
GABOA	gamma aminobetahydroxybutyric acid
gal	gallon
gal	galactose

galv	galvanic, galvanism, galvanized
gang, gangl	ganglion, ganglionic
gangr	gangrene
garg	gargle
GAS, G-A-S	generalized adaptation syndrome
GAS	generalized arteriosclerosis
gastroc	gastronemius
GAT	gas antitoxin
GATB	Government Aptitude Test Battery
GB	gall bladder
GBD	gall bladder disease
G ∉ B days	good and bad days (symptoms subside and recur)
GBH	gamma benzene hydrochloride
GB series	routine series of xray studies
GC	general circulation (systemic)
GC	general condition
GC	glucocorticoid (adrenal cortical hormone)
GC, Gc	gonococcus, gonorrhea
Gca, gca	gonorrhea
g-cal	gram calorie (small calorie)
GCT, GC ∉ T	general care and treatment
GC type	guanine, cystocine type
GCY	gastroscopy
GD, G/D	growth and development
Gd	gadolinium

GDH   glutamic dehydrogenase

GDH   growth and differentiation hormone

gdn   guardian

GDP   guanosine diphosphate

GE   gainfully employed

GE   gastroenteritis

GE   gastroenterology (subspecialty of Internal Med-
                                            icine)

Ge   germanium

g e   gravity eliminated

gel   gelatin, gelatinous

gel quav, gel quavis   in any kind of jelly (pharmacy)
  gelatine quavis

gen   genetics

gen   genitalia

gen   genus

gen cath   Gensini catheter (used in cardiovascular studies)

genet   genetics

gen et sp nov   new genus and species
  genus et species nova

genit   genitalia

gen nov   new genus
  genus novum

geront, gerontol   gerontologist, gerontology

GF   globule-fibril

GF   glomerular filtrate

G forces   acceleration forces

GFR	glomerular filtration rate
GG, γ globulin	gamma globulin
GGE	general glandular enlargement
GGG *gummi guttae gambiae*	gamboge
GH	general health
GH	general hospital
GH	good health
GH	growth hormone
GI	gastrointestinal
GI	globin insulin
gi	gill (¼ pint)
GII	gastrointestinal infection
GIS, GI series	a routine series of films of the gastrointestinal tract
GITT	glucose-insulin tolerance test
GL	greatest length
G/L	grams per liter
Gl	glucinum
GLA	gingivolinguoaxial (tooth planes)
glac	glacial
glau, glauc	glaucoma
glc	glaucoma
glob	globular
glob	globulin
glos dev	glossal deviation

GLTN	glomerulo-tubulo-nephritis
glu, gluc	glucose
glu tol, gluc tol	glucose tolerance
glv	galvanic
glyc	glycerine
glyc	glycerite
glyco	glycogen
GM	General Medicine
gm	gram
gm/l	grams per liter
GMA	gross motor activities
gm/cc	grams per cubic centimeter
GMCD	grand mal convulsive disorder
GMP	guanine monophosphate
GM ⊄ S	General Medicine and Surgery
GMW	gram molecular weight
GNC	General Nursing Council
G/N r, G/N ratio	glucose nitrogen ratio
GOE	gas, oxygen and ether (anesthesiology)
GOK	God only knows
Gold sol	colloidal gold curve solution
GOR	general operating room
GOT	glutamic oxaloacetictransaminase
govt	government
GP	general paralysis

GP	general paresis
GP	General practice, General Practitioner
GP	globus pallidus
GP	guinea pig
[G]p	concentration of glucose in plasma
gp	group
GPB	glossopharyngeal breathing ("frog breathing" done by patients who have had laryngectomies)
GPI	general paresis of the insane
GPM	General Preventive Medicine (subspecialty of Preventive Medicine)
GPT	glutamic pyruvic transaminase
Gp Th	group therapy
GR	gamma roentgen
Gr I AS	grade 1 arteriosclerotic
gr	gamma roentgen
gr	grade
gr	graft
gr	grain
gr	gravity
gr *gravida*	pregnant, with child
gr	great, greater
gr	grill, grilled
gr	gross, grossly
grad	gradient

grad	gradual, gradually
grad	graduate, graduated (one who has completed a prescribed course of study)
grad	graduate, graduated (a vessel marked for measuring liquids)
gran	granulation
grav *gravida*	pregnant, with child
grav	gravity
gravid *gravida*	pregnant
grd, grds	ground, grounds
grp	group
gr wt	gross weight
GS	gastrocnemius soleus (muscle)
GS	General Surgeon
GSA	general somatic afferent
GSE	general somatic efferent
GSH	glutathione (reduced form GSSG)
GSR	galvanic skin response
GSSG	glutathione (oxidized form)
GSW	gun shot wound
GT	gait training
GT	great toe
GT	greater trochanter
GT	group therapy

gt *gutta*	drop (approximately equivalent to one minim, the amount varies with the nature of the liquid)
GTH	gonadotrophic hormone
GTN	glomerulo-tubulo-nephritis
GTO	golgi tendon organ
GTP	guanosine triphosphate
GTR	galvanic tetanus ratio
GTR	generalized time reflex
GTT	glucose tolerance test
gtt *guttae*	drops
GU	genitourinary
[G]u	concentration of glucose in urine
guid	guidance
gutta, guttat *guttatim*	drop by drop (pharmacy)
gutt quibusd *guttis quis busdam*	with a few drops
GV	gentian violet
GVA	general visceral afferent
GVE	general visceral efferent
G ₵ W	glycerine and water
Gyn, gyn	gynecologist, gynecological, gynecology

H *haustus*	a drink
H	flagella (with reference to antigens)
H	Huach (laboratory)
H	height
H	henry (unit of electrical induction)
H	heroin
H	Holzknecht unit
H	husband
H	hydrogen
H	hyoscine (scopalomine)
H	tritium
H^+	hydrogen ion
H^1	light hydrogen
H^2, H^b	deuterium (heavy hydrogen)
H_o	null hypothesis
H_1	alternate hypothesis
H_{11}	extract from human urine containing growth inhibiting substances
H △, H's △	Hesselbach's triangle
H antigens	antigens localized in flagella of motile bacteria
H reflex	Hoffman reflex
H substance	histamine-like substance
H unit	Holzkneckt unit
h	hecto
h	height

h	high
h	horizontal
h	hour
h	hundred
h	Planck's constant
h	quantum constant
h	hypermetropia, hyperopia
h, (h),⒣	hypodermically
HA, H/A	headache (some doctors reserve the use of H/A to mean splitting headache)
H/a	home with advice (emergency room record)
habt *habetur*	let him have
HAGG	hyperimmune antivariola gamma globulin
Hal	halogen
halluc	hallucination
HAP	held after positioning
HA virus	hemadsorption virus
HB, Hʙ	hemoglobin
HB	head backward
HB	heart block
HB	heel to buttock (neurological test)
Hb A∘	hemoglobin determination
hb	hemoglobin
HBD	has been drinking
HBD	hydroxbutyrate dehydrogenase

HBO	hyperbaric oxygen
HBO	oxygenated hemoglobin
HBP	high blood pressure
HC	heel cord
HC	hemoglobin concentration
HC	hemorrhage, cerebral
HC	home call
HC	home care
HC	Hospital Corps
HC	hydrocolator
HC	hydrocortisone
HC	hydrogen ion concentration in M/eq liter
H/C, H ¢ C	hot and cold
HCC	heat conservation center
HCG	human chorionic gonadotrophin
HCl	hydrochloric acid
HCN	hydrocyanic acid
HCO	bicarbonate ion
hct, h'crit	hematrocrit
hct	hundred count
HCVD	hypertensive cardiovascular disease
HD	Hansen's disease (leprosy)
HD	hearing distance
HD	hip disarticulation

HD *hora decubitus*	bedtime
HD	hospital day
HD	hypnotic dosage
hd	head
hd *hora decubitus*	bedtime
HDLW	distance at which a watch is heard with the left ear
HDRW	distance at which a watch is heard with the right ear
HE *hic est*	this is
H ¢ E	hematoxylin and eosin (histology – staining method)
H ¢ E	heredity and environment
H or E	hemorrhages or exudate (eye examination)
He	helium
He *hoc est*	that is
he	head
he	helium
hebdom *hebdomata*	a week
HED *Haut-Einheits Dosis*	unit skin dose
HEENT	head, eyes, ears, nose and throat
HE inj	hyperextension injury
Hem, hem	hemolysis (blood fragility test)

hem	hemorrhage
hem	hemorrhoid
hema	hematuria
hemat	hematocrit
hematem	hematemesis
hematol	hematologist, hematology
hemi	hemiparesis
hemi	hemiplegia
hemo	hemoglobin
hemo	hemophilia
hemo F	hemoglobin free
hemop	hemoptysis
hemorr, hemorrh	hemorrhage, hemorrhagic
her	hernia
hered	hereditary, heredity
hern	hernia, herniated, herniation
Het	heterophil antibody (test)
HETP	hexaethyltetraphosphate (anticholinesterase)
HE virus	human enteric virus
HEW	Health, Education and Welfare
HF	Hageman factor (in blood plasma)
HF	hard filled
HF	head of fetus (pre-natal examination)
HF	head forward
HF	heart failure

HF	high frequency
HF	hot fomentation
Hf	hafnium
hf	half
HFD	high forceps delivery
HF inj	hyperflexion injury
HFO	hard food orientation
Hg *hydroargyrum*	mercury
hg	hectrogram
hg	hemoglobin
Hgb, hgb	hemoglobin
Hbg ∉ Hct	hemoglobin and hematocrit
HGF	hyperglycemia glycogenolytic factor (glucagon)
Hg-F	fetal hemoglobin
HGH	human growth hormone
Hg-Hg Cl	calomel half cells
HGO	hepatic glucose output
HH	hard of hearing
H ∉ H	hemoglobin and hematocrit
HHb	reduced hemoglobin
HHD	hypertensive heart disease
H ∉ HM, H+HM	compound hypermetropic astigmatism, compound hyperoptic astigmatism
HHT, HHTx	head halter traction
HI	hemagglutination inhibition

HI	Hospital insurance
5 HIAA	5 hydroxyindoleacetic acid
HIC	Heart Information Center
Hi CHO	high carbohydrate (diet)
HID syndrome	headache, insomnia and depression syndrome
HIFC	hog intrinsic factor concentrate
H inf	hypodermoclysis infusion
Hin t, Hint test	Hinton test (for syphilis)
Hi Prot	high protein
HIS	Haptic Intelligence Scale
hist	histologist, histolgoy
hist	history
HIT	histamine ion transfer
H→K	hand to knee coordination
HK cells	human kidney cells
HL	half life
HL	hearing loss
HL	Hygienic Laboratory
H/L	hearing loss
Hl	latent hypermetropia
Hl	latent hyperopia
hl	hectoliter
H,L,A negative	heart, lungs and abdomen negative
H) L) O A)	heart, lungs and abdomen negative

HLC	heat loss center
H ₵ L o.k.	heart and lungs normal
HLR	heart-lung resusitation
HM	hand movements
HM	heavily muscled
Hm	manifest hypermetropia (hyperopia)
hm	hectometer
HMC	hyocin-morphine-codeine
HMD	hyalin membrane disease
HMO	heart minute output
HM, WM	heavily muscled, white male
HN	Head Nurse
HN_2	nitrogen mustard
H ₵ N	head & neck
hn *hoc nocte*	tonight
HNLN	hospitalization no longer needed, hospitalization no longer necessary
H ₵ N mot	head and neck motion
HNP	herniated nucleus pulposus
Ho	holmium
H_2O	water
H_2O_2	hydrogen peroxide
HOB	head of bed
hoc (Not an abbreviation)	this

hoc ves *hoc vespere*	this evening, tonight
ho decub *hora decubitus*	bedtime
Hoff refl	Hoffman reflex
Hoff resp	Hoffman response
homatrop	homatropine
homo	homosexual
homolat	homolateral
HOP	high oxygen pressure
HOPE	Health Opportunity for People Everywhere (Government Agency)
HOPI	History of Present Illness
hor	horizontal
hor decub *hora decubitus*	bedtime
hor interm *horis intermediis*	at intermediate hours
hor som *hora somni*	bedtime, hour of sleep
hor un spat *horae unius spatio*	at the end of one hour
hosp	hospital, hospitalize, hospitalization
Hosp Ins	Hospital Insurance
HOT	human old tuberculin
HP	heat production
HP	heel to patella
HP	highly purified

HP	high potency
HP	high power
HP	high pressure
HP	hot packs (wet heat)
HP	hot pad (dry heat, usually electric pad)
HP	hydrostatic pressure
HP	hyperphoria (measurement of squint)
hp	heaping
hp	horse power
H &c P	history and physical (examination)
HP, H &c P	Hodgen and Pearson
H &c P susp trx	Hodgen-Pearson suspension traction
H→P	heel to patella
HPC	history of present complaint
HPD	highly probably drunk
HPF	high power field
/HPF	per high power field
HPG	human pituitary gonadotrophin
HPI	History of Present Illness
HPI (test)	Heston personality Inventory test
HPN, hpn	hypertension
HPP	allopurinal (4 hydroxylpyrazolo 3,4-d pyrimidine)
HPP	history of presenting problems
HR, H/R	heart rate
hr	hour

H reflex	Hoffman reflex
H response	Hoffman response
H substance	histamine-like substance
HRL	head rotated left
HRR	head rotated right
hrs	hours
HS	hamstring
HS	head signs
HS	head sling
HS	heart sounds
HS *hora somni*	hour of sleep (bedtime)
HS	House Surgeon
H/S, H &c S	hemorrhage and shock
hs *hora somni*	hour of sleep (bedtime)
H→S, h→s	heel to shin maneuver
HSA	human serum albumin
HS-Co A	coenzyme in tissue oxidations
hskpg	housekeeping
H substance	histamine-like substance
HT	home treatment
HT	hospital treatment
HT	Hubbard Tank
HT	hypermetropia (ophthalmology)
HT	hypodermic tablet

H & T	hospitalization and treatment
Ht	heart
Ht	total hypermetropia
ht	heart
ht	heat
ht	height
ht	hypodermic tablet
HTB	hot tub bath
HTK	heel to knee (neurological test)
HTP	house, tree, person (free hand drawing test in psychiatry)
HTS	heel to shin (same as heel to knee test – which is done in a different manner by some examiners)
HU	hyperemia unit
hum	humerus
HV	hematocrit value in volumes per cent
HV	hospital visit
HV	hyperventilation
hv _hos vespere_	this evening, tonight
H vs A	home against advice
HVD	half value layer
HW	healing well
H/W, hw	housewife
H wave	Hoffman wave
HWB	hot water bottle

HWOK	heel walking OK
HWP	hot wet pack
hx	history
hx	hypoxanthine
HY	hypermetropia, hyperopia
hy	hysteria
hyd	hydration
hyd	hydraulic
hyd	hydrogenomonas
hyd	hydrostatic
hydro	hydrotherapy
hyd and tur	hydration and turgor
hyg	hygiene
hyp	hyplagesia
hyp	hyperresonance
hyp	hypertrophy
hyper A, hyperact	hyperactive
hypersens	hypersensitive
hyperten	hypertension
hypertens	hypertensive
hypervent	hyperventilation
hypes	hypesthesia
hypn	hypertension
hypnot	hypnotic, hypnotism
hypo	hypodermic

hypo A, hypoact   hypoactive

hys   hysteria, hysterical

hys, hyst   hysterectomy (Example: vag hyst c̄ A c̸ P repair
                              — vaginal hysterectomy with anterior and
                              posterior repair)

Hz   hertz

I	Roman numeral one
I	incisor (permanent)
I	independent (physical function)
I	index
I	induction
I	inspired
I	intensity of magnetism
I	Internal Medicine
I	Internist
I	iodine
I 131, ^{131}I	radioactive isotope of iodine Example: (I 131 uptake radioactive iodine uptake test for thyroid function)
i	incisor (deciduous)
i	insoluble
i	optically inactive
IA	impedance angle
IA	indol-acid
IA	intra-arterial
IA	intra-articular
IA	intra-atrial
IAA	indol-3-acetic acid
IAAR	imidazoleacetic acid ribonucleotide
IAC	Industrial Accident Commission
IAFI	infantile anaurotic idiocy
IAL	ischial apophysialysis (separation of ischial epiphysis)

IASD	interatrial septal defect
IB	inclusion body
IB	index of body build
ib *ibidem*	same place; same authors
I-B	interbody (vertebral)
IBI	intermittent bladder irrigation
ibid *ibidem*	same place; same authors
IBM	isotonic-isometric brief maximum (strengthening technique)
IBU	International Benzoate Unit
IC	color index
IC	inspiratory capacity
IC	inspiratory center
IC	cardiac insufficiency
IC	Intensive Care
IC	intercostal
IC	internal capsule
IC	internal conjugate (obstetric measurement)
IC	interstitial cells
IC	intracerebral
IC	intracutaneous
I č	independent with equipment (physical function)
ICA	internal carotid artery
ICD	internal cervical device

ICF	intracellular fluid
IC fx	intracapsular fracture
ICM	intercostal margin
ICO	initial check out only
↑ ICP	increased intracranial pressure
I,C,PM,M; ICPMM	incisors, canines, premolars, molars (followed by a fraction — the entire permanent dentition formula is shown)
IEA	intravascular erythrocyte aggregation
IEC	intraepithelial carcinoma
IE Ca cx	intraepithelial carcinoma of the cervix
ICR	distance between iliac crests
ICR	intermittent catheter routine
ICS	intercostal space
ICSH	interstitial cell stimulating hormone
ICT	inflammation of connective tissue
ICT	insulin coma therapy
ICT	intermittent cervical traction
ict	icteric, icterus
ict ind	icteric index
ICU	Intensive Care Unit
ID	identification
ID	ill defined
ID$_{\infty}$	infective dose
ID	initial dose
ID	inside diameter

ID	intradermal, intradermally
ID_{50}	median infective dose
I & D	incised and drained, incision and drainage
Id, id *in diem*	during the day
id *idem*	same
id ac *idem ac*	the same as
IDA	iron deficiency anemia
IDM	idiopathic disease of myocardium
IDP	inosine diphosphate
IDT	intradermal typhoid and paratyphoid vaccine
IE *immunitats Einheit*	immunizing unit
IE	inner ear, internal ear
i e *id est*	that is
I ∉ E	internal and external
IER test	Institute of Educational Research (intelligence test)
IF	intermediate frequency
IF	interstitial fluid
if nec	if necessary
IH	infectious hepatitis
IHD	ischemic heart disease
IHSA	iodinated human serum albumin
II	icteric index

I or I	illness or injuries (usually written "No I or I" on history)
IK	immune Korper, immune bodies
IK	interstitial keratitis
Ik	Springler's tuberculin
IKI, I KI	iodine potassium iodide – Lugol's solution
IL	iliolumbar
il	illinium
ILA	insulin-like activity
ill	illusion
ill	illustration, illustrating
illic lag obturat *illico legena obturatur*	stopper the bottle at once
IM	Indicus Medicus
IM	internal malleolus
IM	Internal Medicine (designation of medical specialty)
IM	intramedullary
IM, (IM)	intramuscularly
IMA	Industrial Medicine Association
IME	Independent Medical Examiner, Independent Medical Examination
imit	imitation, imitative
IMM	internal medical malleolus
immat	immature
immed	immediate, immediately
immob	immobile, immobilize

immun	immune, immunize, immunization, immunity
immunol	immunology
IMP	inosine monophosphate
IMP	inpatient multidimensional psychiatric scale
imp	impacted
imp	important
imp	impressed
imp	impression (tentative diagnosis)
imp	improve, improvement, improved
imperf	imperfect
imperf	imperforate
impr	impressed
impr	impression (tentative diagnosis)
impr	improve, improvement, improved
impreg	impregnate, impregnated
impvt	improvement
IMVC	indol, methyl red, Voges-Poskauer, citrate
In	index
In	indium
in	inch, inches
in^3	cubic inch
inadeq	inadequate
inc	increase, increased, increasing
inc	incomplete
inc	inconclusive

inc	incorporated
incid *incide*	cut
incl	include, included, including, inclusive
incoher	incoherent
incompat	incompatible
incont	incontinence, incontinent
incr	increase, increased, increasing
incr	increment
incur	incurable
ind	independent
ind	index
ind	indicate, indicating, indication
Ind Med	Indicus Medicus
ind	indigent
ind	indigo
in d *in die*	in a day, daily
indef	indefinite
Ind H	Industrial Hygiene
indic	indicate, indicated, indication, indicative
indig	indigestion
induc	induction
indur	induration
indus	industrial
Ind Th	Industrial Therapy

ind th	individual therapy
in extrem *in extremis*	at point of death
inf	infancy, infant, infantile
inf	infarct, infarction
inf	infected, infection, infectious
inf	inferior — two separate meanings: 1) below, lower than 2) of less quality
in f *in fine*	finally, at the end
inf	infirmary
inf	information
inf *infunde*	pour in
inf	infusion
infect	infection, infectious
infer	inferior
infl	inflamed, inflammation
infl	influence
infl	influx
infl proc	inflammatory process
inflam	inflamed, inflammation, inflammatory
info, infor	information
infra	(as used in physical therapy) infra red
inf turb	inferior turbinate
infund *infunde*	pour in

Ing, ing	inguinal
INH	isoniazid (chemotherapy for tuberculosis)
inher	inherent
inhib	inhibit, inhibition, inhibitory
INI agent	intranuclear inclusion agent
init	initial
inj	inject, injected, injection (May refer to medication which is injected into tissue or blood vessels or may refer to congestion in tissues from trauma or disease)
inj	injured, injurious, injury
inj enm *injiciatur enema*	give an enema
INK	injury not known
in lb	inch pound
in litt *in litteris*	in correspondence
in loc cit *in loco citato*	in the place cited
innerv	innervate, innervation
innom	innominate
innox	innoxuous
inoc	inoculated, inoculation
inorg	inorganic
in oz	inch ounce
INPRCNS	information processing in central nervous system
in pulm *in pulmento*	in gruel

ins	inches
ins	insulin
ins	insurance
insid	insideous
in situ (not an abbreviation)	a latin phrase meaning natural or normal position
insol	insoluble
insp	inspect, inspection
insp	inspiration, inspiratory
insp'd	inspected
insp'd ∉ p's'd	inspected and passed
inspir	inspiration, inspiratory
Inst, inst	institute, institution, institutional
instab	instability
instn	institution
instr	instructor, instruction
insuff	insufficiency, insufficient
int	intact
int	interest, interesting
int	intermittent
int	internal
Int	Interne
Int	Internist
int	interval
int cib *inter cibos*	between meals

intell	intelligence, intelligent
intercond	intercondylar
intermit	intermittent
intertroch	intertrochanteric
intes, intest	intestine, intestinal
int hist, Int Hist	interval history
Int Noct, int noct *Inter noctem*	during the night
Int Med	Internal Medicine
intracal	intracalvarium
Int Rot, int rot	internal rotation
↑int rot	increased internal rotation (usually beyond normal limits)
↓int rot	decreased internal rotation
int trx	intermittent traction
intub	intubate, intubation
in utero (not an abbreviation)	a latin phrase meaning within the uterus
inv	invalid
inv	inversion, inverted
inv	investigate, investigation
inval	invalid
inver	inversion
invest	investigate, investigation
invet	inveterate
in vivo (not an abbreviation)	a latin phrase meaning within a living body
IO	intraocular

I ∉ O	intake and output (fluid exchange in body)
Io	ionium
IOC	Interne on call
IOFB	intraocular foreign body
IOP	intraocular pressure
IOTA	Information Overload Testing Aid
IP	incisoproximal
IP	initial pressure (opening pressure in lumbar puncture)
IP	inorganic phosphate
IP, I/P	in patient (frequently followed by initials of hospital)
IP	International Pharmacopia
IP	interphalangeal
IP	iso-electric point
Ip	intraperitoneal
I/P	in patient
I/P, I-P	interphalangeal
[I] p	concentration of insulin in plasma
I para	primipara (I in this case is the Roman numeral one)
IPAT	Cattrell's Institute for personality and ability testing anxiety scale
IPD	inflammatory pelvic disease
IPH	infant passive hand
IPMR	Institute of Physical Medicine and Rehabilitation
IPM	infant passive mitt

IPNA	isopropylnoradrenaline
IPPA	inspection, palpation, percussion and auscultation (chest examination)
IPPB	intermittent positive pressure breathing (Bennett respirator)
IPPB/I	intermittent positive pressure breathing, inspiratory
IPPR	intermittent positive pressure respiration
ips	inches per second
IPSP	inhibitory postsynaptic potential
IQ	intelligence quotient
iq *idem quod*	the same as
IR	individual reaction
IR	infra red
IR	inspiratory reserve
IR	internal resistance
IR	internal rotation
IR	intrarectal
Ir	iridium
IRI	iris
IRM	Institute of Rehabilitation Medicine
irreg	irregular
irrig	irrigate, irrigation
irrit	irritable
IRV	inspiratory reserve volume
is	island

IS	interspace
IS	intercostal space
is	isolate, isolation
I substance	inhibitor substance
ISC	interstitial cells
ISD	interatrial septal defect
ISF	interstitial fluid
ISL	inner scapular line
ISL	isoleucine
Is of Lang	Islands of Langerhans
iso	isotropic
isol	isolate, isolated, isolation
isol	isolette (individual isolation unit for infant)
isom	isometric
isom	isometrophic (ophthalmology)
ISP	distance between iliac spines
IST	insulin shock therapy
IT	individual therapy
IT	industrial therapy
IT	intensive therapy
IT	intermittent traction
IT	intertrochanteric (fracture)
I/T	intensity duration
Ita	in such manner
ITh	intrathecal (intraspinal injection)

ITP	idiopathic thrombocytopenic purpura
ITP	inosine triphosphate
ITT	insulin tolerance test
IU	immunizing unit
IU	international unit
IU	intrauterine
[I] U	concentration of insulin in urine
IUD	idoxuridine
IUD	intrauterine (contraceptive) device
IUP	intrauterine pregnancy
IUP,TBCS	intrauterine pregnancy, term birth caesarian section
IUP,TBLC	intrauterine pregnancy, term birth, living child
IUP,TBLI	intrauterine pregnancy, term birth, living infant Usually followed by presentation and sex Example: IUP,TBLI ROA ♀
IV	intervertebral
IV, IV	intravenous
IV	intraventricular
IVC	inferior vena cava
IVCD	intraventricular conduction defect
IVD	intervertebral disc
IVP	intravenous pyelogram
IVSD	interventricular septal defect
IVT	intravenous transfusion
IVU	intravenous urogram
IYS	inverted Y suspensor
IZS	insulin zinc suspension

J	Jewish
J	joint
J	joule
J	journal
J	juice
j	In pharmacy, used at times for the Roman numeral one as the equivalent for i
JAI	juvenile amaurotic idiocy
JAMA	Journal of American Medical Association
Jamar	not an abbreviation — the name of dynamometer
jaund	jaundice
jct	junction
JCAH	Joint Commission on Accreditation of Hospitals
JFS	Jewish Family Service
jentac *jentaculum*	breakfast
JH	juvenile hormone
JJ	jaw jerk (reflex)
JND	just noticeable difference
jour	journal
jrl, jrnl	journal
jt	joint
jug	jugular
jug comp	jugular compression test
jt asp	joint aspiration
junct	junction
juv, juve	juvenile

K	absolute zero
K	cathode
K	constant
K	electrostatic capacity
K	gastric tube
K _kalium_	potassium
K	Kelvin (temperature scale)
K	kidney
K	kilo (metric system prefix meaning 1,000)
K	knee
K−	ionization constant
KA	King-Armstrong units
Ka	cathode
K antigen	capsular antigen
KB splint	knuckle bender splint (dynamic hand splint)
KC	cathodal closing, cathodal closure
kc	kilocycle
K cal	Kilo calorie
KCC	cathodal closing contraction
KCl	potassium chloride
Kcps	kilocycles per second
KCT, KCTe	cathodal closing tetanus
KD	cathodal duration
KDC	cathodal duration contraction

KDT, KD Te	cathodal duration tetanus
Kemo Rx	chemical therapy
Kera	keratitis
kev	kiloelectron volts
kg	kilogram (1,000 grams)
Kg cal	kilogram calorie (large calorie)
kgm	kilogram
kg-m	kilogram meter
kgps	kilograms per second
K hb, K hgb	potassium hemoglobinate
KI	Kronig's isthmus
KI	potassium iodide
kilo	metric prefix meaning one thousand
kilo	kilogram
KJ	knee jerk
Kl, kl	kiloliter
KL bac	Klebs-Loeffler bacillus
Klebs	Klebsiella
km	kilometer
KMEF	keratin, myosin, epidermin, fibrin
$KMNO_4$	potassium permanganate
kmps	kilometers per second
K nail	Kuntscher nail (orthopedics)
KO, K/o	keep on (continue)
KO, K/O	keep open (as in continued intravenous fluids)

KO, K/O	knocked out (unconscious)
KOC	cathodal opening contraction
KP	keratic precipitates
KP *karatio punctata*	keratotic patches
KP	kidney punch test Example: θ KP = negative kidney punch test
Kr	krypton
KS	ketosteroid
17 Ks	17 ketosteroids
K stoff	chloromethyl chloroformate
KU	Kimbel unit
kv	kilovolt
kva	kilovolt ampere
kvcp	kilovolt constant potential
KVP, kvp	kilovolts peak
kw	kilowatt
kw-h, kw-hr	kilowatt hour
K wire	Kirschner wire (orthopedic internal fixation)
kyph	kyphosis

L	coefficient of induction
L	Lambert (unit of light)
L	latin
L	left
L	length
L	lesser
L	lethal
L	Lewisite
L *libra*	pound
L	licensed
L	living
L	lower
L	lumbar
L	Roman numeral 50
(L)	left
L–	Limes death
L I	primary lues (syphillis)
L II	secondary lues
L III	tertiary lues
L_1, L_2, L_3, etc.	lumbar nerves or vertebrae identified by number
L/3	lower third (in reference to long bone)
l	coefficient of induction
l	left
l	length

l	lesser
l	lethal
l *levo*	counterclockwise, to the left
l *libra*	pound
l	licensed
l	light
l	limes
l	living
l	long
l	longitudinal
l	lower
l	lumbar
l	lumen
LA	left angle
LA	left arm
LA	left atrium
LA	left auricle
LA	long acting (medication)
LA	long arm (cast)
L & A	light and accommodation (eye reaction)
L & A	living and active (family history)
La	lanthanum
LAA	left atrial appendage
Lab, lab	laboratory

LAC	long arm cast
lac	laceration
lac $\cancel{c}$ cont	lacerations and contusions
lacr	lacrimal
lact	lactate
lact	lactating
lact (acid)	lactic acid
LAD	lactic acid dehydrogenase
LAE	long above elbow
LAF	latin american female
LAM	latin american male
LAM	left anterior measurement
Lam, lam	laminectomy, laminotomy
lam $\cancel{c}$ fus	laminectomy and fusion
LAO	left anterior oblique
LAP	left arterial pressure
LAP	leucine aminopepidase
LAP	lypholized anterior pituitary
Lap, lap	laparotomy
lar	larynx
laryn	laryngeal, laryngitis
laryngol	laryngologist, laryngology
LAS	left arm sitting (blood pressure taken on left arm while patient sitting)
lat	latent

lat	lateral
lat bend	lateral bending
lat dol *lateri dolente*	to the painful side
lat ₡ loc	lateralizing and localizing (neurology)
lat rot	lateral rotation
lax	laxative
lax	laxity
LB	lateral bending
LB	low back
L ₡ B	left and below
Lb, lb *libra*	pound
lb ap *libra apothecary*	apothecary pound
lb av *libra avoirdupois*	avoirdupois pound
LBB	low back bend, low back bending
LBBB	left bundle branch block
LBBSB, LBB$_s$B	left bundle branch system block
LBBX, LBBx	left breast biopsy examination
LBCD	left border cardiac dullness
LBD	left border of dullness
LBE	long below elbow
LBF	lactobacillus bulgaricus factor
LBH	length, breadth, height
LBP	low back pain

LBP	low blood pressure
lbs *librae*	pounds
LBT	low back tenderness
lb t *libra troy*	pound(s) troy
lc *loco citato*	in the place cited
LCA	left coronary artery
LCB	left costal border
↑**LCB**	upper left costal border, elevated left costal border
↓**LCB**	lower left costal border
L Ch *Licentiate in Chirurgiae*	Licentiate in Surgery
LCCS	low cervical caesarian section
LCL bodies	Levinthal-Coles-Lillie bodies
LCM	left costal margin
LCM	lymphocytic choriomeningitis
LD (bacillus)	lamb dysentery bacillus
LD	laboratory data
LD	lethal dose
LD$_{oo}$	lethal dose
LD	light difference
LD$_{50}$	median lethal dose (lethal for 50% of group tested)
L ¢ D	(eyes react to) light and distance
Ld	laboratory data

Ld	limes — potency of diphtheria toxin
LDA	left dorsoanterior (fetal position)
LDH	lactic dehydrogenase
LDO	local Doctor of Osteopathy
LDP	left dorsoposterior (fetal position)
LDP	lumbodorsal pain
LDS	Licentiate in Dental Surgery
LDT	left dorsotransverse (fetal position)
LDU (brace)	long double upright (brace)
LDUB	long double upright brace
LE	left eye
LE	lower extremity
LE	lupus erythematosus
Le, Le unit	Leonard unit for cathode ray
L/E	lower extremity
lect	lecture, lecturer
LED	lupus erythematosus disseminated
leg	legislation, legislative
Leg Com	legal commitment, legally committed
lenit *leniter*	gently
Lept, lepto	Leptospira
LES	local excitatory state
les	lesion
LET	lineal energy transfer

LEU	leucine
leuc	leucocytes
leuk	leukocytes (german spelling of leucocytes)
levit *leviter*	lightly
L ext, l/ext	lower extremity
LF	left foot
LF	limit of flocculation
LF	low frequency
LF	lineal fracture
Lf	limit of flocculation
lf	left
LFA	left forearm (as in location of allergy sensitivity injections)
LFA	left frontoanterior (fetal position)
LFB	liver, iron and B complex
LFD	least fatal dose (antitoxin)
LFD	low forceps delivery
L-FECT	loose fibroelastic connective tissue
LFP	left frontoposterior (fetal position)
LFT	left frontotransverse (fetal position)
LFT	liver function test
L fx	linear fracture
lg	large
lg	leg
lg	long

lge	large
lgt	ligament
lgts	ligaments
LGV	lyphogranuloma venereum
LH	left hand
LH	lues hereditaria
LH	Prolan-B
LH	luteinizing hormone
LHG	left hand grip
l hr	lumen hour
LHS	left heart strain
L & I	liver and iron
Li	lithium
LICM	left intercostal margin
LIF	left iliac fossa
LIF	left index finger
lig	ligament
lig	ligate
lig	ligature
ligs	ligaments
lim	limit, limitation
lin	linear
lin	liniment
ling	lingual, lingular (pertaining to tongue)
linim	liniment

LIO	left inferior oblique
liq	liquid, liquor
lit	literally
LIVC	left inferior vena cava
LKS	liver, kidneys, spleen
LKS non palp, LKS np	liver kidneys, spleen not palpable
L) K) O S)	liver, kidneys and spleen negative (not palpable)
L M K 0 S T	liver, kidneys and spleen negative, no masses or tenderness (abdomen)
LL	large lymphocytes
LL	left lateral
LL	lid lag (eyes)
LL	long leg (brace or cast)
ll	lid lag (eyes)
LLB	left lateral bending
LLB	long leg brace
LLBCD	left lower border of cardiac dullness
LLBP	long leg brace with pelvic band
LLC, LL cast	long leg cast
LLCC	long leg cylinder cast
LLD	lactobacillus lactis, Dorner factor (vitamin B 12)
LLD, LL discrep	leg length discrepancy
LLE	left lower extremity

LLF	left lateral flexion (neck or back motion)
LLL	left lower lobe (lungs)
LLLE	left lower lid, eye
LLLNR	left lower lobe, no rales
LLOD	lower lid oculus dexter (right eye)
LLOS	lower lid oculus sinister (left eye)
LLQ	left lower quadrant (abdomen)
LLR	left lateral rectus
LLRE	lower lid right eye
LLS	lateral loop suspensor
LLSB	left lower scapular border
LLX	left lower extremity
LM	light microscope
LM	longitudinal muscle
lm	lumen
5 L/M	5 liters per minute
LMA	left mentoanterior (fetal position)
LMCA	left middle cerebral artery
LMCAT	left middle cerebral artery thrombosis
LMCL	left mid-clavicular line
LMD	local Medical Doctor
LMF	left middle finger
LM hormone	lipid mobilizing hormone
LML	left mediolateral (episiotomy)
LML scar w/h	lower mid-line scar with hernia

LML	lower midline
LML scar s̄ h	lower midline scar without hernia
LMN	lower motor neuron
LMNL	lower motor neuron lesion
LMP	last menstrual period
LMP	left mento posterior (fetal position)
LMR	left medial rectus (eye muscle)
LMT	left mento transverse (fetal position)
lmtd	limited
LN	lymph node
LNMP	last normal menstrual period
LOA	leave of absence
LOA	left occiput anterior (fetal position)
loc	local, localized, location
lo cal	low calorie
lo calc	low calcium
loc cit *loco citado*	in the place cited
loc dol *loco dolenti*	painful spot
Lo Cho	low carbohydrates
lo chol	low cholesterol
LOD	line of duty
lo fat	low fat
log	logarithm
LOM	left otitis media

LOM	limitation of motion, limitation of movement
LOM	loss of movement
LOMSA	left otitis media, suppurative, acute
LOMSCh	left otitis media, suppurative, chronic
long	longitudinal
LOP	leave on pass
LOP	left occiput posterior (fetal position)
LOQ	lower outer quadrant
lord	lordosis, lordotic (anterior curve)
LOS	length of stay
LOS	loss of sight
lo salt	low salt
LOT	left occiput-transverse (fetal position)
lot	lotion
lox	liquid oxygen
LP	laboratory procedures
LP	latent period
LP	light perception
LP	lost privileges
LP	low power (microscope)
LP	low pressure
LP	lumbar puncture
LPA	left pulmonary artery
LPA	Licensed Physician's Assistant
LPD	Local Police Department

LPF	leukocytosis-promoting factor
LPF	low power field
LPM	left posterior measurement
LPM	liters per minute
LPMP	last previous menstrual period
LPN	Licensed Practical Nurse
LPO	left posterior-oblique (fetal position)
L Proj	light projection
lps	liters per second
LPT	Licensed Physical Therapist
lpw	lumens per watt
LQ	lower quadrant
LR	latency relaxation
LR	left rotation
L>R	left greater than right
L<R	left less than right
LRF	left ring finger
LRF	liver residue factor
LRMP	last regular menstrual period
LRQ	lower right quadrant (abdomen)
LRR	labyrinthine righting reflex
LS	lateral suspensor
LS	length of stay (in hospital)
LS	liminal sensitivity
LS	lumbosacral

LS	lumbar spine
L ∉ S	liver and spleen
LSA	left sacroanterior (fetal position)
LSB	left scapular border
LSB	left sternal border
LScA	left scapuloanterior (fetal position)
LSD_{25}, LSD^{25}, LSD	lysergic acid diethylamide (hallucinogenic drug — sometimes used in treatment of schizophrenia)
LSK	liver, spleen, kidneys
LSM	lysergic acid morpholide
LSO	left superior oblique
LSO	left salpingo-oophorectomy
LSP	left sacroposterior (fetal position)
L sp	life space
L sp	lumbar spine
LST tract	lateral spinothalamic tract
LST	left sacrotransverse (fetal position)
LSVC	left superior vena cava
Lt, lt	left
Lt, lt	light
LTAF	local tissue advancement flap
LTB	laryngeal-tracheal bronchitis
ltd	limited
LTF	lipotrophic factor
LTH	luteotrophic hormone

LTPP	lipothiamide-pyrophosphate
LTS	long tract sign (neurological test)
lt vent BBB	left ventricular bundle branch block
lt vent BBB occl assoc c̄ SOB	left ventricular bundle branch block occasionally associated with shortness of breath
LU	lung (lobe subscripted)
Lu	lutecium
luc prim *luce primo*	at first light (daybreak)
LUE	left upper extremity
lues I	primary lues (syphillis)
lues II	secondary lues
lues III	tertiary lues
LUL	left upper lobe (lung)
lumb	lumbar
LUOB	left upper outer buttock (site of injection)
LUQ	left upper quadrant (abdomen)
LUOQ	left upper outer quadrant (buttock − location of injection)
LUP	left utero-pelvic junction
LUQ	left upper quadrant (abdomen)
LUSB	left upper scapular border
LV	left ventricle
lv	leave
LVH	left ventricular hypertrophy

LVN	Licensed Vocational Nurse
LVP	left ventricular pressure
L_1 VR, L_2 VR	lumbar ventral nerve root by number
L ⊄ W, L/W	living and well
Lw	laurencium
lx	lower extremity
Ly	Langley (unit of sun's heat)
ly	lying
lym, lymph	lymphocytes
LYS, Lys, lys	lysine

M	macerated
M	male
M	malignant
M	manual
M	married
M	masculine
M	mass
M	massage
M	mature
M	mean
M	media (laboratory)
M	median
M	medical
M	medium
M	membrane
M	memory (association)
M *mentum*	chin
M	meridian (noon)
M	metabolite
M	meter
M	mist
M, *M* *misce*	mix (pharmacy)
M *mistura*	mixture

M	molar (dentistry)
M	molar (refers to concentration of one gram-molecular weight [1 mol] of solute per liter of solution)
M	Monday
M	monocyte
M	morphine
M	mother
M	mucoid, mucous, mucus
M	murmur
M	muscle
M *mutitas*	dullness
M	myopia
M	myosin
M/	mashed
M_1	heart sound at apex
M_1	mitral first sound
M_2; M^2	dose per square meter of body surface
M_1	slight dullness)
M_2	marked dullness) auscultation of heart
M_3	absolute dullness)
M/3	mid-third (In orthopedics the long bones are divided into thirds in order to specifically designate areas of fracture or other injury)
M_8	8th molar
M ∡, Ⓜ ∡	range of motion measurement

M ↻	motion circumduction
m	macerated
m	male
m	manual
m	married
m	masculine
m	mass
m	massage
m	mature
m	media
m	medium
m	membrane
m	memory (association)
m	micro
m *mille, milli*	thousand
m	minim
m	minute
m	modulus
(m), m	by mouth
(m), ⓜ	murmur
m @	melts at (followed by temperature)
m^2	square meter
m^3	cubic meter
√ⓜ , √ⓜ	factitial murmur

MA	Master of Arts
MA	maternal aunt
MA	medical authorization
MA *mentum anterior*	chin anterior (position of fetus)
MA	menstrual age
MA	mental age
MA	meter angle
MA	multiple action
M-A tube	Miller-Abbott tube (gastrointestinal tube)
Ma	masurium
ma	milliampere
MAA	Medical Assistance for the Aged
MABP	mean arterial blood pressure
MAC	maximum allowable concentration
mac	macerate, macerated, maceration (destruction of tissue by action of fluid)
macro	macrocyte, macrocytic (having abnormally large erythrocytes such as are found in pernicious anemia)
macro	macroscopic (visible with the naked eye i.e. no need for enlargement with microscope etc.)
MAF	minimum audible field
mag	magnify, magnification
mag *magnus*	large, larger
maj	major
maj	majority

MAL	midaxillary line
mal	malignant
malad	maladjusted
malig	malignancy, malignant
mal occl	malocclusion (teeth which do not offer proper "bite")
M+AM	myopic astigmatism, compound
MAM, Ma min	milliampere minute
man *manipulus*	handful
man *mane*	morning
mand	mandible, mandibular
manif	manifest, manifested, manifestation
manip	manipulation
manip ↓ anesthesia	manipulation under anesthesia
man pr *mane primo*	early morning
MAO	monoamine oxidase
MAOI	monoamine oxidase inhibition
MAP	minimum audible pressure
MAP	muscle action potentials
MAPS	Make a picture story (psychiatry)
MAR	Main Admitting Room
marg	margin, marginal
MAS	(Taylor) Manifest Anxiety Scale
MaS	milliampere second

mas, masc	masculine
mas pil *massa pilularum*	pill mass (material from which pills are formed)
mass	massage
mass	massive
mast	mastectomy
mast	mastoid
Masters 3	Masters three step
Masters 4+	Masters four step test
MAT	manual arts therapist, manual arts therapy
Mat	maternity
mat	material
mat gf	maternal grandfather
mat gm	maternal grandmother
math	mathematical, mathematics
matut *matutinus*	in the morning
max	maxilla, maxillary
max	maximal, maximum
MB	Marsh-Bender factor
MB	maximum breathing
MB *Medicinae Baccalaureus*	Bachelor of Medicine
MB	methylene blue
MB	muscle balance (eyes)
Mb, mb *misce bene*	mix well

MBC	maximum breathing capacity
MBE	medium below elbow
MBH	maximum benefit from hospitalization
MBH	methylene blue reduced
MBP	mean blood pressure
MBP	melitensis bovine, porcine
McB, McB pt	Mc Burney's point
MC	mass casualty
MC *Master Chirurgiae*	Master of Surgery
MC	Medical Corps
MC	metacarpal
MC	mouth care
M-C	mineralocorticoid (adrenal cortical hormones)
mc	megacycle
mc	millicurie
MCA	middle cerebral artery
MCAS	middle cerebral artery syndrome
MCAT	middle cerebral artery thrombosis
MCC	marked cocontraction
MCD	mean corpuscular diameter
mcd	millicuries destroyed
MCFP	mean circulating filling pressure
mcg, mcgm	microgram
M CH *Master Chirurgiae*	Master of Surgery

MCH	mean corpuscular hemoglobin
mc-h	millicurie-hour
MCHC	mean corpuscular hemoglobin concentration
MC Hgb	mean corpuscular hemoglobin
M Chir *Master Chirurgiae*	Master of Surgery
MCL	mid clavicular line
MCP, MCPH	metacarpal-phalangeal
MCT	manual cervical traction
MCT	mean circulation time
MC USA	Medical Corps United States Army
MC USN	Medical Corps United States Navy
MCV	mean corpuscular volume
MD	manic depressive (psychiatry)
MD	mean deviation
MD	Medical Department
MD	Medical Doctor
MD	mentally deficient
MD	mitral disease
MD	muscular dystrophy
md	median
MDA *mento dextra anterior*	chin to right anterior (fetal position)
MDA	motor discriminative activity
MDCM	Doctor of Medicine and Master of Surgery

m dict *more dicto*	as directed
MDP *mento dextra posterior*	chin to right posterior (fetal position)
MDR	minimum daily requirement
MDS	Master of Dental Surgery
MDT *mento-dextra-transverse*	chin right transverse (fetal position)
ME *Mache Einheit*	unit of measure of radium emanation
ME	Medical Examiner (often refers to the coroner)
ME	member employee (group insurance, etc)
ME	middle ear
Me	methyl
MEA	mercaptoethyl amine
meas	measure, measuring, measurement
MeB	methylene blue
mecano	mechanical therapy
mech	mechanical
MED	median erythrocyte diameter
MED	minimal effective dose
MED	minimal erythema dose
med	medial
med	median
med	medical
med	medicine, medicinal, medication
med	medium

med men	medial meniscus
Medco	medcosonolator
med elig	medical eligibility
Med Sci D	Doctor of Medical Science
med tech	medical technologist, medical technology
MEF	maximal expiratory flow (rate)
meg	megacycle
MEK	methyl ethyl ketone
mel	melena
mem, memb	member
memb, membr	membrane
men, mening	meninges, meningeal, meningitis
menst, menstru	menstrual, menstruate, menstruation
ment	mental, mentation
MEP	mean effective pressure
MEP	motor end plate
mEq	milliequivalent
mEq/L	milliequivalents per liter
MES	muscles in elongated state
MET	methionine
met	metabolic, metabolism, metabolites
met	metal, metallic (foreign body)
met	metallic (chest sounds)
metab	metabolic, metabolism, metabolites
metaph	metaphysis

metas, metast	metastisis, metastasize, metastasizing
M et f pil, *M & f* pil *misce et fiat pilulas*	mix and make into pills
M et f pulv, *M & f* pulv *misce et fiat pulvis*	mix and make into powders
meth	method
meth	methyl
m et n *mane et nocte*	morning and evening
M et sig, *M & * sig *misce et signe*	mix and label
mev, m ev	million electron volts
MF	meat free (diet)
MF	mutton fat (eye)
MF	myocardial fibrosis
M:F	male to female ratio
M & F	mother and father
Mf,	masculine – feminine
mf	microfilariae
mf	millifarad
MFB	metallic foreign body
MFD	minimal fatal dose
mfd	microfarad
MFG	modified heat degraded gelatin
mfg	manufacturing
M flac *membrana flaccida*	Shrapnell's membrane

MF method   membrane and millipore filter method

mfr   manufacture, manufacturer

MFRL   maximum force at rest length

MFS   Minnesota Follow-up Study

MF sol   merthiolate formaldehyde solution

M ft,   make a mixture (pharmacy)
  mistura fiat

MFT   muscle function test

MFU   medical follow up

Mg   magnesium

mg,   milligram (1/1000 gram)

mg%   milligrams per cent (per hundred parts)

mg el   milligram element

MGF   maternal grandfather

mgh, mg h, mg/hr, mg-hr   milligrams per hour

MGM   maternal grandmother

mgm   milligram (1/1000 gram)

mgm/100 ml   milligrams per 100 milliliters

mgmt   management

mgr   manager

$MgSO_4$ magnesium sulfate

mgt   management

MH   marital history

MH   melanophore hormone

MH   menstrual history

MH	mental health
MH	mid-half (flow 25% to 50% rate of forced expiratory spirogram)
MH	military history
mh	millihenry
MHB	maximum hospital benefit
MHD	metahydran
MHD	minimum hemolytic dose
MHRI	Mental Health Research Institute
MH virus	virus murine (hepatitis virus)
MI	mental illness
MI	mitral insufficiency
MI	myocardial infarction
MI	myocardial ischemia
mic, micro	microscope, microscopic
microbiol	microbiologist, microbiology
microgtts	microdrops
MID	minimum infective dose
mid	middle
mid sag	midsagittal
MIF	maximal inspiratory flow (rate)
MIFR	maximal inspiratory flow rate
MIF tech	merthiolate iodine formaldehyde technic
MIL	mother in law
mil	milliliter (1/1000 liter)

mil   military

millirem   milliroentgen equivalents, man

millirep   milliroentgen equivalents, physical

mil TB   miliary tuberculosis

min   mineral

min   minim (drop)

min   minimal, minimum

min   minor

min   minute

/min   per minute

MIO   minimal identifiable odor

misc   miscellaneous

mist   mixture (pharmacy)
  mistura

mit   send
  mitte

mit insuf   mitral insufficiency

mitt   send
  mitte

mitt sang   bleed (seen in old writings – refers to the
  mitte sanguinum   bleeding of patients as a cure for disease)

mitt tal   send such
  mitte tales

MJT   Meade Johnson tube

MK   main kitchen

MK cells   monkey kidney cells

mkd, mkdly   marked, markedly

MKG	meter kilogram
mks	meter kilogram second
ML	maximum (cardiac bulge) to left
ML	marked latency
ML	midline
mL	millilambert
ml	marked latency
ml	midline
ml	milliliter (1/1000 liter)
MLA *mento laevo anterior*	chin left anterior (fetal position)
MLD	metachromatic leukodystrophy
MLD	minimal lethal dose
MLD_{50}, mld_{50}	minimal lethal dose for 50% of test animals in a series
MLF	medial longitudinal fasciculus
MLP *mento laevo posterior*	chin left posterior (fetal position)
MLT *mento laevo transverse*	chin left transverse (fetal position)
MM	medial malleolus
MM	mucous membrane
mM	millimole
mm	medial malleolus
mm	mucous membrane
mm	muscles
MMF	maximal midexpiratory flow

mmg	millimicrogram
mmHg	millimeters of mercury
mml	micromilliliter
mmm	micromillimeter
MMPI	Minnesota Multiphasic Personality Inventory
mmpp	millimeters of practical pressure
mm/sec	millimeters per second
mm str	muscle strength
MMT	manual muscle test
MN	mononuclear
MN	motor neuron
Mn	manganese
mN	millinormal
mn	midnight
MND	minimal necrosing dose
MO	mineral oil
MO	minute output
Mo	mode
mob, mobil	mobility
MOD	mesial occlusal distal (planes of tooth)
mod	moderate
mod praesc *modo praescripto*	in the manner prescribed, as directed
mol	molecular, gram molecule
moll *mollis*	soft

mol wgt, mol wt	molecular weight
MOM	milk of magnesia
MO-MOM, MO Ȣ MOM	mineral oil and milk of magnesia
mon, mono	monocytes
mono	mononucleosis
mor dict *moro dicto*	in the manner directed
morph	morphine
morph	morphological, morphology
mort	mortality
mos	months
mosm, mOsm	milliosmol
MP	menstrual period
MP	mental petition
MP *mentum posterior*	chin posterior (fetal position)
MP	mesiopulpal
MP	metacarpal phalangeal (hand)
MP	metatarsal phalangeal (foot)
MP	moist pack
MP	motor power
MP	mucopolysaccharide
6 MP	6 mercaptopurine
MPC	maximum permissible concentration
MPD	maximum permissible dose
MPH	Master of Public Health

mph	miles per hour
MPI	Multiphasic Personality Inventory
MPL	maximum permissible level (or limit)
MPM	Murphy-Punch maneuver (test)
MPN	most probable number
MPS	mucopolysaccharides
MR	maximum (cardiac bulge) to right
MR	may repeat (Example: MR x 1 = may repeat one time)
MR	medicine radiation
MR	medicine reaction
MR	medical release
MR	mental retardation
Mr	metabolic rate
MR	methyl red
M/R	may repeat
M R	maintenance and repair
mr	milliroentgen
MRA	melody, rhythm, accent
MRD	minimal reacting dose
mrd	millirutherford
mrep	milliroentgen equivalents, physical
mrhm	milliroentgen per hour at one meter
MRL	medical records librarian
MR 0, MR 0̸	no masses or rebound

MRU	minimal reproductive units
MRVP	methyl red Voges-Proskauer medium
MS	Master of Surgery
MS	mitral sounds
MS	mitral stenosis
MS	morphine sulfate
MS	multiple sclerosis
MS	muscle shortening
MS	muscle strength
M/S	meters per second
Ms	murmurs
Ms	muscles
M/s^2	meters per second squared
MSA	mine safety appliance
msec	millisecond
MSG	monosodium glutamate
MSH	melanocyte stimulating hormone
MSL	midsternal line
MSN	Master of Science in Nursing
Msp, Msp, m sp	muscle spasm
MSRPP	Multidimensional Scale for Rating Psychiatric Patients
mss	massage
MST	mean survival time
MSTh	mesothorium

MSTI	multiple soft tissue injuries
M stim	muscle stimulation
M str	muscle strength
MT	manual traction
MT	medical technologist (MT ASCP = Registered medical technologist, American Society of Clinical Pathologists)
MT *membrana tympana*	tympanic membrane (ear drum)
MT	metatarsal
MT	microtherm
MT	muscle test
MT	music therapy
MT_6	mercaptomerin
M/T	(no) masses or tenderness
M ¢ T	monilia and trichomonas
Mt	metatarsal
MTAD *membrana tympana auris dextra*	tympanic membrane, right ear
MTAS *membrana tympana auris sinistra*	tympanic membrane, left ear
MTAU *membrana tympana auris unitas*	tympanic membranes, both ears
MTD	Monroe tidal drainage
MTP	metatarsal phalangeal
MTR-0	no masses, tenderness or rebound
M T } 0 R	no masses, tenderness or rebound

MTR	Meinicke turbidity reaction
MTR	Music Therapist, Registered
MTRG, MTR/G	masses, tenderness, rebound or guarding
M L T 0 K R S	no masses, tenderness or rebound and liver, kidneys and spleen not palpable
MTT	mean transit time (blood through heart and lungs)
M tuberc	Mycobacterium tuberculosis
MTV	metatarsus varus
mu	mass unit
mμ*	millimicron
MU	maternal uncle
MU	mouse unit (laboratory)
Mu	Mache unit (measure of reaction of emanation)
muc	mucilaginous
muc	mucoid, mucous
muco-pur	mucopurulent
mμEP*	millimicron equivalents, physical
mult	multiple Example: mult cont abras = multiple contusions and abrasions
mult inj	multiple injuries
multip	multipara
mus, musc	muscle, muscular
mus-lig, musc ligt	musculoligamentous

*μ is the symbol for micron (greek letter mu) but often looks like u when hand written and therefore is included here.

mut	mutilated, mutilation
MV	meningovascular
MV	microvolt
MV	minute volume
mv	microvolt
MVA	motor vehicle accident
MVC	maximum voluntary contraction
MVV	maximum voluntary ventilation
MW	microwave
MW	molecular weight
MWD	microwave diathermy
mx	minims (drops)
my	mayer
my	myopia
myco	mycobacterium
mycol	mycology
myel	myelin
myel	myelocyte
myel	myelogram
myel sched	myelogram scheduled
myo, myocard	myocardial, myocardium

N	Avogadro's number
N	nasal
N *natus*	born
N	negative
N	negro
N	Neisseria
N	nerve
N	neural
N	neurologist, neurology (designation of medical specialty)
N	neuter
N	neutral
N	neutrophil
N	Newton
N	nitrogen
N	none
N	non-malignant
N	noon
N	normal
N	number (total)
N I, N II or N 1, N 2	cranial nerves by number
n	index of refraction
n	nano (one billionth of a unit)
n	nasal
n	nerve

n	neutron charge
n	normal
$_2$n	index of refraction, diploid number
NA	negro adult
NA	no abnormalities
NA	not applicable
NA	not available
NA	numerical aperture (microscope objective)
N/A	negro adult
N/A	no abnormalities
N/A	not applicable
N/A	not available
N ¢ A	normal and active (reflexes, use, etc)
Na *natrium*	sodium
Na Cl	sodium chloride
NAD	nicotinamide adenine dinucleotide
NAD	no active disease
NAD	no acute distress
NADH	nicotinamide adenine necleotide dehydrogenase
NAF	negro adult female
NaHCO	sodium bicarbonate
NAI	no active inflammation
NAI	no acute infection
NAM	negro adult male

NAR	no action required
NAS	no added salt (diet)
nat	national (referring to national origin)
nat	native
nat	nature, natural
NB	newborn
NB	northbound (description of position of vehicle in traffic accident)
NB *nota bene*	note well
NB	nuclear bag
Nb	niobium
NBM	nothing by mouth
NBO	non bed occupant
NBS	National Bureau of Standards
NC	neck complaints
NC	negro child
NC	nitrocellulose
NC	no card (clinic registration card or insurance identification card)
NC	no change
NC	no charge
NC	no complaint
NC	non-contributory
NC	normocephalic
NC	Nurse Corps

N/C	nerves and circulation
N/C	no change
N/C	no charge
N/C	no complaint
N ⊄ C	nerves and circulation
NCA	neurocirculatory asthenia
NCD	no congenital deformities
NCDC	National Communicable Disease Center
NCI	naphthalene creosote iodoform powder
NCO	no complaints offered
NCOA	National Council on Aging
NCV	nerve conduction velocity
NCVS	nerve conduction velocity studies
ND	nasal deformity
ND	neutral density
ND	not dictated
ND, N/D	not done
Nd	neodynium
Nd	symbol for refractive index
NDV	Newcastle disease virus
NE	new employer (on insurance forms)
NE	not enlarged
Ne	neon
NEA	no evidence of abnormality
NEC	not elsewhere classified

NEC	not elsewhere coded
NEC	no essential change
nec	necessary
NED	no evidence of disease
NEFA	non-esterified fatty acids
neg	negative
nem	Nahrung's Einheit Milch
nema	nematode
Nemb, nemb	nembutal
neo (Not an abbreviation)	a prefix meaning new
neo, neoars	neoarsphenamine
neonat	neonatal, neonatorum
neopl	neoplasm
NEP	no evidence of pathology
neph	nephritis
ner, nerv	nervous, nervousness
neut	neuter
neut	neutral, neutralize
neut	neutrophil
NF	National Formulary
NF	National Foundation (formerly NFIF)
NF, N/F	negro female
NFD	no family doctor (seen on Emergency Room records)
nfe	non-ferrous extract

NFIF	National Foundation for Infantile paralysis (now National Foundation)
NFP	no family physician (seen on Emergency Room records)
NFTD	normal, full term delivery
NFTSD	normal, full term, spontaneous delivery
NG	nasogastric
NG	no good
NG fdgs	nasogastric feedings
NG tube	nasogastric tube
N-Ger	Neurological Geriatrics
NGR	narrow gauze roll
NH	neurologically handicapped
NH	Nursing Home
NH_3	ammonia
NH_4Cl	ammonium chloride
NHS	National Health Service
Ni	nickel
NIA, nia	niacin
nil (not an abbreviation)	nothing
NIMH	National Institute of Mental Health
NIP	no infection present
NIP	no inflammation present
NIS	no inflammatory signs
NIT	National Intelligence Test
nitro	nitroglycerine

NKA	no known allergies
NL	normal libido
NL	normal limits
nl *non licet*	not permitted, not lawful
nl *non liquet*	not clear
NLRB	National Labor Relations Board (handles Industrial Accident cases)
NLC ∉ C, NL C/Cl	normal libido, coitus and climax
NLD	nasolacrimal duct
NLN	National League of Nursing
NLNE	National League of Nursing Education
NLP	no light perception
NM	negro male
NM	neuromedical, neuromedicine
NM	neuromuscular
NM	nitrogen mustard
N/M	negro male
N/M	neuromuscular
N ∉ M	nerves and muscles
nm, n ∉ m *nocte et mane*	night and morning
NMI	no middle initial
NMN	nicotinamide mononucleotide
NMN	no middle name
NMTS	neuromuscular tension state

NN	neonatal
NN *nomen novum*	new name
NN	Nurses Notes
N:N	azo group
nn	neonatal
nn	nerves
nn *nomen novum*	new name
NNC	Navy Nurse Corps
NND	New and Nonofficial Drugs
NNR	New and Nonofficial Remedies
NNR	not necessary to return (to clinic or office)
NO, N_2O	nitrous oxide
No	nobelium
no	number
noc	night
no compl	no complaints
no compl	no complication
noct *nocte*	night
noct	nocturia
noct maneq *nocte et maneque*	night and morning
no ess abn	no essential abnormalities
NOK	next of kin

nom dub *nomen dubium*	doubtful name
nom nov *nomen novum*	new name
nom nud *novem nudem*	name without a designation
noncontrib	non-contributory
non rep *non repetatur*	do not repeat
nonspec	nonspecific
nontend	nontender
NOP	not otherwise provided for
NOPHN	National Organization of Public Health Nursing
nor, norm	normal
normoceph	normocephalic (normal head)
nor Na Cl	normal saline solution (isotonic with blood i.e. 0.9%)
NOS	not on staff (physician from outside hospital staff)
NOS	not otherwise specified
nos	numbers
nov *novum*	new
nov n *nomen novum*	new name
nov sp *novum species*	new species
noxt	nights
NP	nerve palsy

NP	neuropsychiatric, neuropsychiatry (designation of medical specialty)
NP	new patient
NP	not palpable
NP	nucleoplasmic (index)
NP	nucleoprotein
NP	nursing procedure
Np	neptunium
*$\aleph$ p, $\mathcal{N}$ p	high energy phosphate bond
NPC	near point of convergence (vision)
NPD	Niemann-Pick's Disease
NPE	no palpable enlargement
NPH	neutral protamine Hegedorn insulin
NPI	Neuropsychiatric Institute
NPN	non protein nitrogen
NPO *nil per os*	nothing by mouth
NPOW	not prisoner of war
NP polio	nonparalytic poliomyelitis
NPT	normal pressure and temperature
NR	nerve root
NR	neutral red
NR	nonreactive
NR	nonrebreathing

*symbol for energy — this is not an N but is included here because when handwritten, it often looks like an N.

NR	no report
NR	no respirations
NR	no results
NR	no return (indicating no further appointments necessary)
NR	normal range
NR	normal reaction
NR	not remarkable
nr	near
nr *non repetatur*	do not repeat
NRC	National Research Council
NRC	normal retinal correspondence
NRI	nerve root involvement
NRI	nerve root irritation
NRM	normal range of motion
NRN	no return necessary
NRO	Narcotics Rehabilitation Officer
NROM	normal range of motion
NRS	normal rabbit serum
NS	needle shower (physical therapy)
NS	nervous system
NS	neurosurgeon, neurosurgery (designation of medical specialty)
NS	neurosurgical
NS	normal saline

NS	normal serum
NS	no show (did not keep appointment)
NS	not seen
NS	not specified
N/S	normal saline
N/S	normal serum
N-S	Northrupp-Sierra (prosthesis)
Ns	nerves
NSA	no significant abnormalities
nsa	no salt added (diet)
NSAD	no signs of acute disease
NSC	National Safety Council
NSC	Not Service Connected (injury or illness not connected with duties in the Armed Forces or industrial service)
NSCCA, NSCC A	National Society for Crippled Children and Adults
NSD	normal spontaneous delivery
NSE	normal saline enema
N s̊ E	nausea without emesis
NSF	National Science Foundation
NSFTD	normal, spontaneous, full term delivery
NSI	no signs of infection
NSI	no signs of inflammation
NSM	neurosecretory material
NSPCC	National Society for Prevention of Cruelty to Children

NSPF	not specifically provided for
NSR	normal sinus rhythm (heart)
NSS, NS sol	normal saline solution
NSS	normal size and shape
NSSL	normal size, shape and location
NSS ȼ M	normal size, shape and mobile (uterus)
N surg	neurosurgical, neurosurgeon, neurosurgery
NSX	neurosurgical examination
nsy	nursery
NT	nasotracheal
NT	neotetrazolium
NT	nontender
NT	normal temperature
NT	nose and throat
NT	no test, not tested
Nt	niton
N ȼ t, N ȼ thr	nose and throat
NTG	nitroglycerine
NTO	not thrown out (of vehicle)
NTP, NT ȼ P	normal temperature and pressure
nt wt	net weight
nuc, nucl	nucleus, nucleated
nullip	nulliparous
NV	naked vision
NV	nonveteran

NV	not verified
N ¢ V	nausea and vomiting
N or V	nausea or vomiting
Nv	naked vision
NVDC-O, NVDC O	no nausea, vomiting, diarrhea or constipation
NW	not weighed (premature infant)
NWB	no weight bearing (orthopedic orders)
NWB	non-weight bearing (cast or brace)
NYD	not yet diagnosed
ny hor *nystagmus horizontalis*	horizontal nystagmus
ny rot *nystagmus rotatorius*	rotatory nystagmus
ny und *nystagmus undulans*	undulant nystagmus
ny vert *nystagmus verticalis*	vertical nystagmus

O	negative, nil, no, none
O	occipital, occiput
O *octarius*	pint
O *oculus*	eye
O	ohne Hauch
O	old
O	opening
O	oral, orally
O	orthopedic
O	other
O	output
O	oxygen (more properly written O_2)
O	zero
(O),	oral, orally
O̶	negative, nil, no, none
O_2	oxygen
O_2	both eyes
O_3	ozone
O_2 sat	oxygen saturation
ō *octarius*	pint
o, ⓞ	oral, orally
o	orthopedic
ȯ, ō	negative, nil, no, none

O
P

ō (reversal)   no reversal

OA   occiput anterior (fetal position)

OA   old age

OAA   Old Age Assistance

OAA   oxaloacetate

O antigens   body antigens, somatic antigens

OAS   Old Age Security

OASI   Old Age and Survivors Insurance

OASP   organic acid soluble phorphorus

OB***   observed value

OB, Ob   obstetric, obstetrical, obstetrician

ob   he (or she) died
  obiit

ob   obstetric, obstetrician, obstetrical

OBD   organic brain disease

OBG, Ob-Gyn   obstetrics and gynecology, obstetrician and gyne-
                                  cologist (designation of medical specialty)

obj   object, objective

obl   oblique

OBS   organic brain syndrome

obs   obsolete

obs, obst   obstetric

obst   obstipation

obst   obstruct, obstruction obstructive

obstet   obstetric

OC   occlusocervical

OC	office call
OC	oxygen consumed
O ¢ C	onset and course
oc *opere citato*	in the work cited
occ	occasion, occasional, occasionally
occ	occipital, occiput
occ	occupation
occ△	occipital triangle
occas	occasional, occasionally
occip	occipital, occiput
occip F, occip-F	occipitofrontal
occip-F HA	occipitofrontal headache
occl	occlusion
OCC Th	occupational therapist, occupational therapy
occup	occupation, occupational
occup	occupies, occupying
oct *octarius*	pint
OD	occupational disease
OD *oculus dexter*	right eye
OD	Officer of the Day
OD *omni die*	every day, daily
OD	open drop (method for giving general anesthesia)
OD	optical density

OD   Doctor of Optometry

OD   Doctor of Osteopathy

OD   outside diameter

OD   overdose

ODA   right occiput anterior (fetal position)
  occipitodextra anterior

OD'd   overdosed

ODP   right occiput posterior (fetal position)
  occipitodextra posterior

ODT   right occiput transverse (fetal position)
  occipitodextra transversa

OE   orthopedic examination

OE   inflammation of external ear
  otitis externa

O ∉ E   observation and examination

oesoph   oesophageal, oesophagoscopy, oesophagus

OF   occipitofrontal

OF   optic fundi

ofc   office

off   official

O-FHA, OF-HA   occipitofrontal headache

OF PF   optic fundi and peripheral fields

OF rad   occipitofrontal radiation

OG (stain)   orange-green stain

OGTT   oral glucose tolerance test

OH   occupational health

OH *omni hora*	every hour
OH	hydroxyl group
OH-	hydroxyl ion
17 OHCS	17 hydyroxycorticosterioids
OHD	organic heart disease
OHI	ocular hypertension indicator
OI	opsonic index
OI *otitis interna*	inflammation of inner ear
OIC	Officer in Charge
oint	ointment
OJ	orange juice
OK	all right, approved, correct
OKN	optokinetic nystagmus
OL, ol *oculus laevus*	left eye
ol *oleum*	oil
ol oliv *oleum olivae*	olive oil
ol res *oleum resini*	castor oil
OLA *occiput laevo anterior*	occiput left anterior (fetal position)
OLP *occiput laevo posterior*	occiput left posterior (fetal position)
OLR	Otology, Laryngology and Rhinology (designation of medical specialty)

OLT   occiput left transverse (fetal position)
  occiput laevo transversa

OM   occipitomental (fetal position)

OM   Occupation Medicine (special field of Preventive
                                           Medicine)

OM   every morning
  omni mane

OM   Osteopathic Manipulation

OM   inflammation of middle ear
  otitis media

OMAC   otitis media, acute, catarrhal

OMAS   otitis media, acute, suppurating

OMCA   otitis media, catarrhal, acute

OMCC   otitis media, catarrhal, chronic

OMChS   otitis media chronic, suppurating

omn bih   )
omn 2 hor   )   every two hours
omn 2 h   )
  omni bihora

omn hor   every hour
  omni hora

omn noc, omn noct   every night
  omni nocte

omn quad hor   every quarter hour
  omni quadrante hora

omn sec hor)
omn 2 hor   )   every two hours
omn 2 h   )
  omni secunda hora

OMPA   otitis media, purulent, acute

OMPA   octamethyl pyrophosphoramide

OMPC, OMPCh	otitis media, purulent, chronic
OMT, OM/T	osteopathic manipulation treatment
ON	occipito-nuchal
ON *omni nocte*	every night
ON	Optic nerve
O–N, O→N	zero to neutral (function test)
oncol	oncological, oncology
ONP	operating nurse procedure
O ∉ O	off and on
o/o	on account of
OOB	out of bed
OOD	Officer of the Day
OOLR	Ophthalmology, Otology, Laryngology and Rhinology (designation of medical specialty)
OOP	out of plaster Example: AP lat lt leg OOP = anteroposterior and lateral xrays of left leg out of plaster
OOW	out of wedlock
OP	occipitoparietal
OP	occiput posterior (fetal position)
OP	opening pressure (lumbar puncture)
OP	operating, operation
OP	operative procedure
OP	ophthalmic, ophthalmology
OP	osmotic pressure
OP	other than psychotic

OP, O/P	out patient
O ∉ P	ova and parasites Example: Stool spec for O & P = stool specimen for ova and parasites
op *opus*	work
OPC	out patient clinic
op cit *opere citato*	in the work cited, in the work quoted
OPD	optical path difference
OPD	out patient department
OPD	out patient dispensary
oper	operate, operating, operation, operator
Oph, oph, ophth, ophthal	ophthalmologist, ophthalmogy (designation of medical specialty)
oph, ophth, ophthal	ophthalmia, ophthalmic
oph, ophth, ophthal	ophthalmoscope
OPL	osmotic pressure of the proteins in lymph
OPP	osmotic pressure of the plasma colloids
opp	opposed, opposing, opposite, opposition
op reg	operative region
oprg, oprtg	operating
Opt	optical, optician, optics
Opt	optometrist
opt	optical, optician, optics
opt	optimum
OR	open reduction
OR	operating room

OR	Own Recognizance (release from "medical hold" or from jail on own promise to return)
O-R	oxidation reduction
or xl	oriented as to time
or x2	oriented to time and place
or x3	oriented as to time, place and person
ORA	occiput right anterior (fetal position)
orch	orchitis
ord	order, ordered
ord	orderly
OR en	oil retention enema
OR ₵ F	open reduction and fixation (orthopedics)
org	organ, organic, organism
ORIF, OR c̄ IF	open reduction with internal fixation
orig	origin
Or J	orange juice
oro	mouth
ORP	occiput right posterior (fetal position)
ORS	Orthopedic Surgery (designation of medical specialty)
orth, ortho, orthop	orthopedic, orthopedist
orthot	orthotonus
OS _oculus sinister_	left eye
OS	occipitosacral (fetal position)
os	mouth

os	osmium
OSD	outside doctor (one not on staff)
OSFT	outstretched finger tips (used in evaluation of forward flexion in back examination Example: OSFT to midtibia)
OSN	Off Service Note
OSS	over shoulder strap
osteo	osteoarthritis
osteo	osteomyelitis
osteo	osteopathy
osteo	osteopathology
osteoarth	osteoarthritis
osteocart	osteocartilaginous
OT	objective test (psychology)
OT	occupational therapist, occupational therapy
OT	office treatment
OT	old terminology
OT	old tuberculin
OT	orthopedic technician
OT	orthopedic treatment
OT, Ot	Otolaryngologist, Otolaryngology (designation of medical specialty)
OT, ot	Otologist, otology
OT***	total oxygen content
OTA test	orthotolindine arsenite test (test for blood in urine)

OTC	over the counter (drugs sold without prescription)
OTC	oxytetracycline
OTD	organ tolerance dose
oto, otol	otologist, otology
OTR, OT reg	Occupational Therapist, Registered
OTS	Occupational Therapy Student
OU *oculus unitas*	both eyes
OU *oculus uterque*	each eye
OV	office visit
ov *ovum*	egg
OVR	Office of Vocational Rehabilitation
OW	off work
OW	out of wedlock
OX	orthopedic examination
Ox, oxy	oxygen
oxy	oxymel
OCSP	Orthopedic Examination, special
oz	ounce
oz ap	apothecary ounce
oz t	ounce troy

P   para, parous Refers to the number of previous
                           pregnancies that have gone to the period of
                           viability
                           Examples: P O = nullipara (none)
                                       P i = unipara (one)
                                       P ii = bipara or secundipara
                                       P iii = tripara etc.

P   parental

P   part

P   partial performance (functional ability grading)

P   passive

P   percentile

P   perceptual

P   pharmacopeia

P   phenolphthalein

P   a pin or dowel which holds a crown in place
                           (dentistry)

P   phosphorus

P   pint

P   plasma

P   point

P   pole

P   by weight
  pondere

P   population

P   position

P   positive

P   post-prefix meaning after or following

P   posterior (behind, in back of)

P	post partum (on delivery room sheet)
P	presbyopia (ophthalmology)
P	pressure
P	private
P	probability
P	produces
P	protestant
P	protein
P	proximal
P	psychiatrist, psychiatry (designation of medical specialty)
P	psychosis
P	pulmonary
P	pulse
P *punctum proximum*	near point (of vision)
P	pupil
P	pureed
P	P waves — a part of electrocardiograph pattern
p	page
p	papilla
p	para, parous
p	part
p	passive
p *per*	by, through, by means of

p	pica
p	pin, dowel (dentistry or orthopedics)
p	pint
p	plasma
p	pole
p	point
p	poor
p	post (prefix meaning after, following)
p	probable
p	pupil
p	pureed
P_1, P_2 etc	parental generation by number i.e. first parental generation, second generation, etc.
P+	poor plus
P_2	pulmonary second sound
P_3	proximal third (long bones are divided into thirds for accuracy in describing location of injury or lesion)
P_3	luminous flux
P_{32}	radioactive isotope of phosphorus
PA	paralysis agitans
PA	passive aggressive (personality)
PA	paternal aunt
PA	pathology
PA	peridural artery
PA	pernicious anemia

PA	phosphoarginine
PA	pineapple
PA	postaural
PA	posteroanterior (position of xray views)
PA	prolonged action (drugs)
PA	proteolytic activity
PA	psychoanalysis, psychoanalyst
PA	pulmonary artery
PA	pulpoaxial
Pa	proactinium
pa	pathology
P/A	percussion and auscultation
P/A	position and alignment
P ∉ A	percussion and auscultation
P ∉ A	position and alignment (fractures)
P ∉ A	present and active (reflexes)
PAA *poliomyelitis anteria acuta*	acute anterior poliomyelitis
Paa, paa *parti affectae applicandus*	apply to the affected parts
PABA	para aminobenzoic acid
PAC	phenacetin, aspirin, caffeine
PAC	premature auricular contraction
PaCO	arterial carbon dioxide pressure
PAD	phenacetin, aspirin, deoxyephedrine

p ae   equal parts
   partes aequales

PAF   paroxysmal auricular fibrillation

PAH   para-aminohippuric acid

PAL   posterior axillary line

palp   palpable, palpation

palp   palpitation (forcible pulsation of the heart, per-
                              ceptible to the patient, usually with increase in
                              frequency, with or without irregularity)

palpi   palpitation, palpitations

PAM   crystalline penicillin G in 2% aluminum mono-
                              sterate

2 PAM   pyridine-2-aldroxine

PAN   periarteritis nodosa

PAP   passive agressive personality (psychiatry)

PAP   primary atypical pneumonia

PAP   pulmonary alveolar proteinosis

pap   nipple-like
   papilla

Pap in canthus   papilloma inner canthus

Pap sm   Papanicolaou smear (test for cancer cells)

PAR   post-anesthesia recovery room

para (not an abbreviation)   parous (refers to the number of previous preg-
                              nancies that have gone to the period of viability)

para   paraparesis

para   paraplegia

par aff   part affected

para C, para c   paracervical

para L	paralumbar
parapsych	parapsychology
para T	parathoracic
parasym div	parasympathetic division (autonomic nervous system)
par aff	part affected
paravert	paravertebral
parent	parenteral, parenterally
parox	paroxysmal
PARR	post-anesthesia recovery room
part	parturition
part ae, part aeq *partes aequales*	equal parts
part dol *partes dolentes*	painful parts
part vic *partis vicibus*	divided doses
PARU	post-anesthesia recovery unit
PAS	phosphatase acid serum
PAS	para-aminosalicylate
PAS	periodic acid Schiff hemotoxylin stain
PAS	Professional Activities Study
PASA	para-aminosalicylic acid
P'ase	phosphatase
pass	passive
Past	pasteurella
PAT	paroxysmal auricular tachycardia

pat	patella
pat	patient
pat gf	paternal grandfather
pat gm	paternal grandmother
path	pathogen, pathogenic, pathogenesis
path	pathological, pathologist, pathology
pat med	patent medicine
path fx	pathological fracture
pat T	patellar tenderness
PB	powder board
PB	pressure breathing
PB	pressure, barometric
P $\bar{c}$ B	pain and burning (with urination)
Pb	phenobarbital
Pb, pb	phonetically balanced
Pb *plumbum*	lead
Pb	presbyopia
PBC	point of basal convergence
PBE	Perlsucht bacillen emulsion
PBI	protein bound iodine
PB I^{131}	protein bound radioactive iodine
PBZ, Pbz	pyrabenzamine
PC	panting center
PC	pelvic cramps

PC	phone call
PC	phosphocreatine
PC	pneumotoxic center
P closure	plastic closure
PC	polycentric
PC *pondus civile*	avoirdupois weight
PC	posterior cervical
PC	posterior chamber (eye)
PC	present complaint
PC	presenting complaint
PC	privilege card
PC	pulmonary circulation
pc	per cent
pc	piece
pc *post cibum*	after meals
P-C	phlogistic corticoid
P-C syndrome	posterior cervical syndrome
P-C syndrome c̄ ch tens	posterior cervical syndrome with much tension
PCA	passive cutaneous anaphylaxis
PCA	posterior cerebral artery
PCA	posterior communicating aneurysms
Pcb *puncta convergence basalis*	near point of convergence (ophthalmology)
PCc	periscopic concave

PCF   prothrombin conversion factor

PCH   paroxysmal cold hemoglobinuria

pCO_2 arterial carbon dioxide pressure (or tension)

pcpt   perception

pcpt   precipitate, precipitation

pcs   preconscious (psychiatry)

pct   per cent

PCT   plasmacrit test (for syphilis)

PCU   Progressive Care Unit

PCV   packed cell volume (hematology)

PCW   Paul C. Williams (brace or exercises)

P Cx   periscopic convex

PD   interpupillary distance

PD   papilla diameter

PD, PD °°   paralyzing dose, paralytic dose

PD   pediatrics (designation of medical specialty)

PD   percentage difference

PD   Doctor of Pharmacy
  Pharmaciae Doctor

PD   phenyldichlorarsine

PD   potential difference (psychiatry)

PD   prism diopter

Pd   palladium

pd   by the day
  per diem

pd   period

pd, p-d	prism diopter
PDA	pediatric allergy (subspecialty of pediatrics)
PDA	patent ductus arteriosis
PDB	paradichlorobenzene
PDC	pediatric cardiology (subspecialty of pediatrics)
PDC	preliminary diagnostic clinic
PDC	private diagnostic clinic
PDE	paroxysmal dyspnea on exertion
PDR	Physician's Desk Reference
PDR	progress direct report
pdr	powder, powdered (more often written pulv or pwd)
PDRB	Permanent Disability Rating Board
PE	pelvic examination
PE	percentage of estimated normal value
PE	physical education
PE	physical examination
PE	point of entry (penetrating wounds)
PE	present examination
PE	probable error
PE	pulmonary embolism, pulmonary embolus
P/E	point of entry (penetrating wound)
Pe	pressure on expiration
p e *per exemple*	for example
PEA, PE↓A	pelvic examination under anesthesia

PED	pediatrics, pediatrician
PED	post-entry day (hospital notes showing number of days since patient was admitted to the hospital)
PED	postexertional dyspnea
P Ed	physical education
Ped	pediatrics
ped	pedangle (sit up in bed with legs dangling over the side of the bed)
ped	pedestrian
ped ed	pedal edema
PEF	peak expiratory flow
PEG	pneumoencephalogram, pneumoencephalograph
pen	penicillin
pen	penis
pend	pendulous
penic	penicillin
pens	pension
Pent	Pentothal
PEP	phosphoenolpyruvate
per (Not an abbreviation)	through, by means of
per	perineal
per	period, periodic
per	person
Perc	percodan
perf	perfect, perfected
perf	perforated, perforating, perforation

peri	perineal, perineum
periorb	periorbital
periph	peripheral
periumb	periumbilical
PERLA	pupils equal and react to light and accommodation
perm	permanent
per op emet *peracta operatione emetici*	when action of emetic is over
per os (Not an abbreviation)	a latin phrase meaning by mouth
perp	perpendicular
per pad	perineal pad (Kotex etc)
PERRLA	pupils equal, round, regular and react to light and accomodation
pers	person, personal
pers	personality
persp	perspiration
pert	pertinent
pert	pertaining to
per unc	period of unconsciousness
pet	petrolatum Example: liq. pet. = liquid petrolatum (mineral oil)
petich	petichiae
PETN	pentaerthritol tetranitrate
PF	past findings
PF	peak flow

PF	peripheral fields (ophthalmology)
PF	pertinent findings
PF	plantar flexion
PF	push fluids
Pf	Pfeifferella
pf	point of fusion (ophthalmology)
PG	post graduate
6 – PG	6 phosphogluconate
PG	pressure of gas
pg	pregnancy, pregnant
PGA	pteroylglutamic acid
PGE	posterior gastroenterostomy
PGF	paternal grandfather
PGM	paternal grandmother
PGP	progressive general paralysis
PGR	psychogalvanic response
PH	past history
PH	personal history
PH	physical history
PH	Public Health (subspecialty of Preventive Medicine)
Ph	pharmacy
Ph	phenyl
pH	symbol for expression of concentration of hydrogen ions (degree of acidity)
PHA	phenylalanine

Phar, phar	pharmacist, pharmacy
phar	pharyngeal, pharyngitis, pharynx
Phar B	Bachelor of Pharmacy
Phar C	Pharmaceutical Chemist
Phar D	Pharmaceutical Doctor
Phar G	Pharmacy Graduate
pharm	pharmaceutical
phar	pharmacopoeia
pharm	pharmacist, pharmacist
pharyn	pharyngeal, pharyngitis
PhB	Bachelor of Philosophy
PHC	post hospital care
Ph B	Bachelor of Philosophy
PHC	post hospital care
PhD	Doctor of Philosophy
PHD	pin hole disc (ophthalmology)
phen, phenobarb	phenobarbital
PHI	phosphohexose isomerase
PHK (cells)	postmortem human kidney cells
PhM *Pharmaciae Magister*	Master of Pharmacy
PHN	Public Health Nurse
phos	phosphatase
phot	photophobia
PHS	Public Health Service

P Hx	past history
Phys	physician
phys	physical
phys	physics
Phys Dis	physical disability
Phys Ed	physical education
Phys Med	Physical Medicine (medical specialty)
physio	physiotherapy
physiol	physiological, physiology
phys sol	physiological (saline) solution
phys ther	physical therapist, physical therapy
PI	International Pharmacopoeia
PI	personal injury
PI	ponderal index
PI	post injury
PI	present illness
PI	pressure on inspiration
PI	proactive inhibition
PI	protamine insulin
P/I	post injury
PICA	posterior inferior cerebellar artery
PID	pelvic inflammatory disease
PID	post-inertia dyskinesia
pig, pigm	pigmented
PIIS	posterior inferior iliac spine

pil *pilula*	pill
PIP	probable intrauterine pregnancy
PIP	proximal interphalangeal (crease or joint)
pit	pituitary, pituitrin
PITR	plasma iron turnover rate
PK (reaction)	Prausnitz-Küstner reaction
PK	psychokinesis
pK	dissociation constant
PKU	phenylketonuria — a metabolic disease affecting mental development
PL	(degree of) perception of light
pl	place
pl	plasma
pl	plate
pl	pleural
pl	plexus
pl	plural
plac praev	placenta praevia
pleth	plethoric
pls	please
PM *post mortem*	after death
PM, pm *post meridian*	afternoon
PM	mean pressure (of a gas)

PM	Physical Medicine (designation of medical specialty)
PM	polymyositis
PM	presystolic murmur (heart)
Pm	promethium
[61] PM	radioactive isotope of promethium
PM clinic	physical medicine clinic
PM lividity	post-mortem lividity
PM splint	posterior molded splint
PMA	positive mental attitude
PMA test	Primary Mental Abilities test
PMB	polymorphonuclear basophilic leucocytes
PMB	post-menopausal bleeding
PMC	Physical Medicine Clinic
PMD	private medical doctor
PME	polymorphonucelar eosinophilic leucocytes
PMH	past medical history, previous medical history
PMI	past medical illness
PMI	petition of mental illness
PMI	point of maximum impact
PMI	point of maximum impulse
PMI	point of maximum intensity
PML	pulmonary microlithiasis
PMN	polymorphonuclear neutrophils (leucocytes)
PMN	polymorphonucleotides

PMNL	polymorphonuclear leucocytes
PMP	previous menstrual period
PMR, PM ∉ R	Physical Medicine and Rehabilitation
PMRS, PM ∉ RS	Physical Medicine and Rehabilitation Service
PMS	poor miserable soul
PMS	postmenopausal syndrome
PMS	pregnant mare's serum
PMSG	pregnant mare's serum gonadotrophin
PMT	premenstrual tension
PN	percussion note
PN	peripheral nerve
PN	post nasal
PN	post nausea
PN	practical nurse
PN	psychoneurology, psychoneurotic
P/N	post nausea
P ∉ N	psychiatry and neurology
Pn	pneumatic (splint or tourniquet)
pn	pain
pn	pneumonia
pn, pnth, pnthx, pnx	pneumothorax
PNA	pentosenucleic acid
PNAvQ	positive-negative ambivalent quotient (psychology – psychiatry)
PNC	penicillin

PND	paroxysmal noctural dyspnea
PND	post nasal drainage, post nasal drip
PNE	pneumoencephalogram
PNE	practical nurse education
pneu	pneumatic (cuff or tourniquet)
pneu	penumonia
PNF	proprioceptive neuromuscular fasciculation
pnfl	painful
PNH	paroxysmal nocturnal hemoglobinuria
PNI	peripheral nerve injury
PNP	pneumoperitoneum
PNPR	positive-negative pressure respiration
PNPR	positive-negative pressure respirator
PNS	peripheral nervous system
pnt	point
pnts	points
PNX, pnx	pneumothorax
PO	parieto-occipital
PO	percentage of observed value
PO *per os*	by mouth
PO	phone order
PO, P/O, P-O	postoperative
Po	polonium
po	predominant organism

PO_2, pO_2	oxygen pressure
PO_4	phosphate
POA	primary optic nerve
POB	penicillin oil beeswax
POC	products of conception
pocill *pocillum*	small cup
pocul *poculum*	cup
POD	postoperative day
Pod D	Doctor of Podiatry
POE	pediatric orthopedic examination
POE, P of E	portal of entry, point of entry (penetrating wound)
POF	position of function
POF	pyruvate oxydation (alkalinity of solution)
pOH	hydroxyl concentration (alkalinity)
pois	poison, poisonous
polio	poliomyelitis
poly, polys	polymorphonuclear luekocytes
pond *pondere*	by weight
P Op, P-op	postoperative
pop	popliteal
pop	population
poplit	popliteal
port	portable

Pos, pos	position
Pos, pos	positive
poss	possible, possibility
POSS	proximal over shoulder strap
post	posterior
post	prefix meaning after, following
post	post mortem examination (after death) autopsy, necropsy
post mortem	
post aur *post aurem*	behind the ear
post gangl	postganglionic
postop	postoperative
post part	postpartum (obstetrics)
postred, post-red	postreduction
post tib	posterior tibial
post traum	post trauma
pot	potassium
pot	potential
pot	potion
pot *potus*	a drink
potass	potassium
POV	privately owned vehicle
POW	prisoner of war
powd	powder, powdered
POX	point of exit (penetrating wound)

PP *paralysis progressiva*	progressive paralysis
PP	partial pressure
PP	pellagra preventive
PP	peripheral pulses
PP *per pro*	instead of
PP	placement problem
PP	plaster of paris
PP	post partum (after delivery)
PP	post prandial (after meal)
PP	presenting problem
Pp *punctum proximum*	near point (ophthalmology)
pp	post prandial
pp	pages
pp	pedal pulses
pp	pluripara (a woman who has had two or more children)
PPA	palpation, percussion and auscultation
ppa *phiala prius agitata*	having first shaken the bottle
PPA pos	phenylpyrubic acid positive (phenylketonuria present)
PPB	positive pressure breathing
PPBS	postprandial blood sugar
PPC	Professional Performance Committee
PPC	progressive patient care

PPCF	plasma prothrombin conversion factor
PPD	permanent partial disability
PPD	purified protein derivative (test for tuberculosis)
Ppd, ppd	packs per day (cigarette consumption)
PPF, P-P factor	pellagra preventive factor (niacinamide)
PPGIR	psychophysiological gastrointestinal reaction
PPH	past pertinent history
PPLO	pleuropneumonia-like organisms
ppm	parts per million
ppn	penicillin
PPO	pleuropneumonia organisms
PPR	posterior primary rami
P Pr	prosthetic-group removing enzyme
pps	pulses per second
Ppt	pneumoperitoneum
ppt	precipitate
pptd	precipitated
ppt LBP	precipitates low back pain
pptn	precipitation
PPT vib pos	pin prick, touch, temperature, vibration and position (neurology)
PQ	permeability quotient
PQ	personal quality (psychiatry)
PR	percentile rank
PR	perfusion rate

PR	peripheral resistance
PR	phenol red
PR	pressoreceptor
PR	progress report
PR	prolonged release
PR	prosthetic group removing enzyme
PR	public relations
PR	pulse rate Example: PR=VR means pulse rate equals ventricular rate
PR, Pr *punctum remotum*	far point of accomodation (eyes)
Pr	praseodymium (element of rare earth group)
Pr	presbyopia (ophthalmology)
Pr	prism
Pr	proctologist, proctology (designation of medical specialty)
Pr	propyl
pr	pair
p r, p rec	per rectum
PRA	progressive resistance to arms (progressive resistance exercises to upper extremities)
prac	practice
pract	practical
prand *prandium*	dinner, meal
p rat aetat *pro ratione aetatis*	in proportion to age
PRD	partial reaction of degeneration

PRE	progressive resistance exercises
prec	preceding
precip	precipitate, precipitation
precord	precordial
pred, prednis	prednisone, prednisolone
pref	prefer, preference
prefd	preferred
preg	pregnant
pregang	preganglionic
pregn	pregnant
prelim	preliminary
prelim diag	preliminary diagnosis
prem, premie	premature infant
preop, pre-op	preoperative
prep	prepare
prepd	prepared
prepn	preparation
pres	pressure
preserv	preserve, preservation
press	pressure
prev	prevent, prevention
prev	previous
prev hx	previous history
prevoc	prevocational
PR ex, pr ex	progressive resistance exercises

PRH	past relevant history
prim	primary
prim diag	primary diagnosis
primip *primipara*	first pregnancy
prin	principal
prin	principle
priv	private
priv	privilege
PRL	progressive resistance to leg (physical therapy)
PRN, prn *pro re nata*	as necessary, as indicated, as circumstances may require
PRO, pro	protein
prob	probable, probably, probability
prob	problem
proc	procedure
proc	proceeding
proc	process
Proct, proct	proctologist, proctology (designation of medical specialty)
procto	proctoclysis
prod	produces, product
pro dose (Not an abbreviation)	for a dose
prof	profession, professional
prof	professor
prog	program

prog	progress, progressive
prog, progn	prognosis
progr	progress
proj	project
proj	projection (xray)
prol	prolong, prolonged
PROM	passive range of motion
pron	pronate, pronated, pronation
pro rat aetat *pro ratione aetatis*	in proportion to age
pros	prostate
pros, prosth	prosthesis, prosthetist
PROT, prot	protein
PROT, Prot	protestant
prothrom	prothrombin
pro time, proth time	prothrombin time
pro us ext *pro uso externo*	for external use
prox	proximal
PRPP	5 phosphoribosyl pyrophosphate
PRR	pulse repetition rate
PRU	unit of peripheral resistance
PS	paraspinal, paraspinous
PS	physical status
PS	present symptoms

PS	Plastic Surgeon, plastic surgery (designation of medical specialty)
PS	point of symmetry
PS	postscript
PS	pulmonary stenosis
PS	serum from pregnant woman
Ps	pseudomonas
P ∉ S, p ∉ s	permanent and stationary (disability rating)
Ps An	psychoanalysis, psychoanalyst
PS closure	plastic surgery closure
PSE	point of subjective equality (psychiatry)
psf	pounds per square foot
PSH	past surgical history
PSI *per secundum intentionem*	by second intention (healing of wound)
PSI	posterior sagittal index
psi	pounds per square inch
PSI apparatus	Problem Solving Information Apparatus
psia	pounds per square inch absolute
psig	pounds per square inch gauge
PSIS	posterior superior iliac spine
PSL	potassium, sodium chloride, sodium lactate solution
PSMA	progressive spinal muscular atrophy
PSNS	parasympathetic nervous system
P sol	partly soluble

P/sore	pressure sore
PSP	posterior spinous process
PSP, psp	postsynaptic potential
PSS	progressive systemic sclerosis
PST	perceptual span test
PSt *punctum sternalis*	sternal puncture
P+st	poor plus start
P subst	protein substance
P surg	plastic surgeon, plastic surgery
PSW	psychiatric social worker
psy, psych	psychiatric, psychiatrist, psychiatry
psy, psych	psychologist, psychology
psychoan	psychoanalysis
psychopath,	psychopathic, psychopathological
psychopathol	psychopatholgical, psychopathology
psychophys	psychophysics
psychosom	psychosomatic
psychother	psychotherapy
PTA	plasma thromboplastin antecedent
PTA	prior to admission
PTAP	purified toxoid precipitated by aluminum phosphate
p'tase	phosphatase
PTB	patella tendon bearing (brace)
PTC	patient to call

PTC	patient to clinic
PTC	Pharmacy and Therapeutics Committee
PTC	phenylthiocarbamide
PTC	plasma thromboplastin component
PTD	permanent total disability
PTD	personality trait disorder (psychiatry)
PTE	pretibial edema
pterg	pterygium
PTF	plasma thromboplastin factor
PTH	parathyroid hormone (parathormone)
PTH	prior to hospitalization
Pth	pneumothorax
PTL	plasma thyroxin level
PTMD	pupils, tension, media, discs (eyes)
PTMFD	pupils, tension, media, fundus, discs
PTO	Perlsucht tuberculin original
PTO	please turn over (page, etc)
PTP	post tetanic potentiation
PTR	patella tendon reflex
PTR	patient to return
PTR	Perlsucht tuberculin rest
P trx	pelvic traction
PTSA	patient's surface area
PTT	prothrombin time
PTU	propylthiouracil

PTWTKG	patient's weight in kilograms
P Tx, ptx	pelvic traction
P tx, p tx	pelvic traction
PU	paternal uncle
PU	pregnancy urine
PU	prostatic urethra
Pu	plutonium
pub	pubic
PUD	possible ulcer, duodenal
Pu D	pulmonary diseases (medical specialty, sub-specialty of internal medicine)
puerp	puerpium
pul	pulmonary
pulm *pulmentum*	gruel
pulm	pulmonary, pulmonic
pulv *pulvis*	powder
pulv	pulverize
PUMS	permanently unfit for military service
punct	puncture
PUO	pyrexia of undetermined origin
pur	purulent
PV	paravertebral
PV	peripheral vascular
PV	plasma volume

PVA	polyvinyl alcohol
PVB	paravertebral block
PVB	premature ventricular beats
PVC	polyvinyl chloride
PVC	pulmonary venous capillary
PVC	premature ventricular contractions
PVD	peripheral vascular disease
PVD c̄ ASO	peripheral vascular disease with arteriosclerosis obliterans
PVE	prevocational evaluation
PVM	pneumonia virus of mice
PVN	paraventricular nuclei
pvn *per vias naturales*	by natural ways
PVP	polyvinyl pyrolidone
PVR	pulmonary vascular resistance
PVT	paroxysmal ventricular tachycardia
pvt	private
PW	pinwheel (neurological testing for sensation)
pw	pin worms
PWB	partial weight bearing
PWB	Paul Williams brace
pwd	powder
P/X	point of exit (bullet etc)
Px	physical examination
px	pneumothorax

px	prescription
px	prognosis
px	point of exit (bullet, missile etc)
pyr	pyridine
PZA	pyrazinamide
PZI	protamine zinc insulin

Q	coulomb
Q *quaque*	each, every
Q	quantity, quantitative
Q	quarter
Q	quartile
Q	question
q *quaque*	each, every
q	quarter
$Q°$, $Q2°$, or $q°$, $q2°$ etc.	every hour, every two hours, etc.
Q', $Q2'$, or q', $q2'$, etc.	every hour, every two hours, etc.
Q_1, Q_2, etc.	first (lowest) quartile, second quartile, etc.
Q_{10}	temperature quotient
Q test	Quick's test
q am	every morning
QAP	quinine, atabrine, plasmochin treatment
QB	whole blood
QBV	whole blood volume
QCIM	Quarterly Cumulative Index Medicus
qd *quaque die*	every day
QED *quod erat demonstradum*	that which is demonstrated
QF	concentration of substance in blood
qh *quaque hora*	every hour

Q
R

q 2h, q3h, etc   every two hours, every three hours, etc

QID, qid   four times daily
 quater in die

QL, ql   as much as you please, amount desired
 quantum libet

qlty   quality

qm   every morning
 quaque mane

Q-M sign   Quenu-Muret sign

qn, q noc   every night
 quaque nocte

QNS, qns   quantity not sufficient

Q O$_2$ oxygen consumption

QOD, qod   every other day
 quaque otra die

QOH, qoh   every other hour
 quaque otra hora

QON, qon   every other night
 quaque otra nocte

QP   Quanti-Pirquet reaction

qp   amount desired
 quantum placet

qqh   every quarter hour
 quaque quarta hora

qr   quarter, quarterly

QRS   ventricular complex on electrocardiogram

QRZ   wheal reaction time
 Quaddel Resorption Zeit

QS, qs   sufficient quantity
 quantum sufficiat

q s ad *quantum sufficiat ad*	sufficient quantity to (make a specific amount)
Q's angle	Quatrefages angle (parietal angle)
Q's sign	Quant's sign
Q's test	Quick's test
Q-S test	Queckenstedt-Stookey test
q suff *quantum sufficiat*	quantity sufficient
QT	blood volume per unit time
QT	Quick's test
qt	quantity, quantitative
qt	quart
qt	quiet
qt dx	quantities duplex
qtr	quarter, quarterly
quad	quadrant
quad	quadriceps
quad	quadriplegia, quadriplegic
quad ex	quadriceps exercises
qual	quality
qual anal	qualitative analysis
quant	quantity
quant suff	quantity sufficient
quar	quarantine
quer	querulous
quest	question, questionable

quinq   five
  quinque

quint   fifth
  quintus

quint, quint N   trigeminal nerve
  nervus quintus

quor   of which
  quorum

quot   quotient

quot   every day
  quotidie

quot   as often as needed
  quoties

quot o s   as often as needed
  quoties opus sit

qv   quantity you desire
  quantum vis

qv   which see (reference in literature)
  quode vide

R	gas constant
R	organic radical
R	radioactive mineral
R	radiologist, radiology
R	radius (bone in forearm)
R	Rankine (temperature scale)
R	rare
R	raw
R	Réaumur
R	rectal, rectally
R	Reiz (stimulus)
R	remote point of convergence (eyes)
R	residue, residuum
R	resistance (electrical)
R	resistant (to disease or to antibiotic therapy)
R	respiration
R	respiratory (tract or system)
R	respond, response
R	review
R	Rickettsia
R, (R)	right
R	roentgen (unit), roentgenologist, roetgenology
R	rough (bacterial colonies)
R	rounded
R	"side chain" in amino acid formulas

R	rub
R test	reductase test
r	rare
r	ratio
r	round, rounded
−R	negative Rinnes test (hearing test)
+R	positive Rinnes test
(R)	rectal
(R), R	registered trade mark
R_1, R#1 (anesthesia risk)	good risk
R_2, R#2 (anesthesia risk)	fairly good − minimal heart or lung condition, or possibly an older patient
R_3, R#3 (anesthesia risk)	poor − pathology which makes anesthesia a poor risk or the surgery contemplated may be severe
R_4, R#4 (anesthesia risk)	very poor risk − not expected to survive
RA	reading age
RA	repeat action (drugs)
RA	residual air
RA	rheumatic arthritis (acute rheumatic arthritis is rheumatic fever) usually written RF
RA	rheumatoid arthritis (atrophic form of arthritis deformans which is a chronic disease of unknown etiology causing deformity and loss of function of one or more joints)
RA	right angle
RA	right arm
RA	right atrium
RA	right auricle

Ra	radium
Ra, ra *radix*	root
Ra, ra	radial, radius
RAA	right atrial appendage
rac	racemic (a compound which is optically inactive)
RAD	radiation absorbed dose
Rad	radiologically, radiologist, radiology
Rad	radiation therapy
rad	radian
rad	radiate, radiating
rad	radical (referring to operative procedure)
rad	radicular, radiculitis
rad/s	radians per second
Rad Ther	radiotherapist, radiotherapy
RAI	radioactive idodine
RAIU, RAI uptake	24 hour radioactive iodine uptake
RAM	rapid alternating movements
RAM	right anterior measurement
ramb	rambling (description of speech)
RAO	right anterior oblique
ran	random
RAR	right arm, resting (seen with blood pressure reading)
RAS	reticular activating system

RAS, RA-S	right arm, sitting (seen with blood pressure reading)
RB	Red Blanket (designates definite emergency.) In some hospitals, patients needing special, rapid transportation and care, a red blanket or a sheet with a red stripe are placed over the patient on the guerney to indicate the urgency for immediate attention.
Rb	rubidium
RBBB	right bundle branch block
RBBSB, RBBsB	right bundle branch system block
RBBX	right breast biopsy examination
RBC	red blood cells, red blood corpuscles
RBC	red blood count
RBD	right border of dullness
RBE	relative biological effectiveness (regarding radiation)
RBF	renal blood flow
RC	conditioned response
RC	red cell
RC	Red Cross
RC	respirations ceased
RC	respiratory center
RC	Roman Catholic
RC	root canal (tooth)
RCA	right coronary artery
RCD	relative cardiac dullness
RCF	relative centrifugal force

RCM	right costal margin
RCO	aliphatic acyl radical
RCT	Rorschach content test
RC TNTC	red cells too numerous to count
RD	radial deviation
RD	reaction of denervation
RD	respiratory disease
RD	retinal detachment
Rd, rd	rutherford (unit of radioactivity)
rd	reading
R & D	research and development
RDA	right dorsoanterior (fetal position)
Rd A	reading age
RDB	research and development board
RDE	receptor destroying enzyme
Rdm	readmission
RDP	right dorsoposterior (fetal position)
RdQ	reading quotient
RDT	right dorsotransverse (fetal position)
RE	radium emanation
RE	rear end (accident)
RE	rectal examination
RE	resistive exercises
RE	reticuloendothelium
RE	right eye

re	regarding
R/E, R ¢ E	round and equal (pupils)
R/E	rear end (accident)
R/E	rectal examination
R↑E	right upper extremity
R↓E	right lower extremity
readm	readmission, readmit
REC	rear end collision
rec *recens*	fresh
rec	recessive (genetics)
rec	recipe (pharmacy)
rec	recommend
rec	record
rec	recreation
rec	recovery
rec	recur, recurrence, recurrent
re ch	recheck
recd	received
recip	recipient
recog	recognize, recognition
recomm	recommend, recommendation
recond	recondition
reconstr	reconstruction
recryst	recrystalize

rect	rectify, rectified
recumb	recumbent
recur	recurrence, recurrent
RED	Research and Experimental Department
red	reduce, reduction
red in pulv *reductus in pulverum*	reduced to powder
redig in pulv *redigatur in pulverum*	reduce to powder
re-ed	re-educate, re-education
re-eval	re-evaluate, re-evaluation
re-ex	re-examination
ref	refer, referred, reference
ref →	refer to
Ref Dr	referring doctor
ref ind	refractive index
refl	reflect, reflection
refl	reflex
Ref Phys	referring physician
REG	radiographic encephalogram (scintogram)
REG	radiation exposure guide
Reg	registered
reg	regime, regimen
reg	region
reg	regular
regen	regenerate, regeneration

reg rhy	regular rhythm
reg R ⊄ R	regular rate and rhythm
reg umb	umbilical region
rehab, rehabil	rehabilitation
REL	rate of energy loss
RELE	resistive exercises, lower extremities
rel	related
rel	relative, relatively
R ⊄ LLQ	right and left lower quadrants
REM	rapid eye movements (in dreaming state)
REM	roentgen equivalent man
rem	remarks
rem	roentgen equivalent man
remg	remaining
remit	remittent
ren	renew
ren sem *renovetur semel*	renew once
REP, rep	roentgen equivalent physical
REP, ReP	retrograde pyelogram
rep *repetatur*	repeat
rep	report
rept	repeat
rept	report
reptd	reported

REO	respiratory enteric orphan
RER	renal excretion rate
RES	reticuloendothelial system
Res	Resident (physician, surgeon)
Res	residence (nurse's residence or doctor's residence)
res	research
res	resect, resection
res	reserve
resched	reschedule, rescheduled
resid	residual
resist	resistance, resistive
resp	respiration, respiratory, respirator
resp	respond, response
resp → ext stimuli	responds to external stimuli
resp → pn stim	responds to painful stimuli
resp → nox stim	responds to noxious stimuli
resp → verb stim	responds to verbal stimuli
resp	responsible
REST	regressive electroshock treatment
Ret	retarded
ret	retained
ret	retarded
ret	retention
ret	reticulocyte
ret	retina

ret	retire, retired
ret	return
retic	reticulocyte
retr	retract, retracted, retraction
REUE	resistive-exercises to upper extremities
rev	reverse
rev	review
rev	revolution
Rev of Sym	review of symptoms
Rev of Sys	review of systems
re-x	re-examination
RF	relative flow (rate)
RF	reticular formation
RF	rheumatic fever
RF	rheumatoid factor
RFA	right frontoanterior (fetal position)
rfd	referred
RFP	request for payment
RFP	right frontoposterior (fetal position)
RFR	refraction
RFS	rapid frozen section (laboratory)
RFS	relaxing factor system
RFT	right frontotransverse (fetal position)
RGE	relative gas expansion

RH	right hand, right handed Example: RHCM = right handed caucasian male
Rh	Rhesus factor (positive or negative blood factor component)
Rh	Rhipicephalus
Rh	rhodium
rh	rhonchi
RHC	respirations have ceased
RHD	relative hepatic dullness
RHD	rheumatic heart disease
rheo	rheostat
RHF	right heart failure
RHG	right hand grip
rheum	rheumatic, rheumatism
rheum	rheumatoid
rheum fev	rheumatic fever
rheum ht dis	rheumatic heart disease
rhin	rhinitis, rhinologist, rhinology
Rhiz	Rhizobium
RI	radioisotope
RI	refractive index (ophthalmology)
RI	respiratory illness
RI	retroactive inhibition (psychiatry)
RIB	riboflavin
RICM	right intercostal margin
RID	ruptured intervertebral disc

RIF	right iliac fossa
RIF	right index finger
RIO	right inferior oblique
RIP	reflex inhibiting posture
RIPP	resistive intermittent positive pressure
RISA	radioiodinated human serum albumin
RIVC	right inferior vena cava
RIVD	ruptured intervertebral disc
RKG	radioelectrocardiogram
RKY	roentgen kymography
RL	reduction level (reciprocal of respiratory quotient)
RL	Reiz limen (stimulus)
RL	resting length
RL	right lateral
RL	Ringer's lactate (intravenous solution)
RL coarse rales	RL_1 few coarse rales RL_2 moderate coarse rales RL_3 many coarse rales
Rl medium rales	Rl_1 few medium rales Rl_2 moderate medium rales Rl_3 many medium rales
rl fine rales	rl_1 few fine rales rl_2 moderate fine rales rl_3 many fine rales
R/L	right/left
$R > L$	right greater than left, right more than left
$R < L$	right less than left

R ¢ L	right and left
RLA	react to light and accommodation
RLB	right lateral bending
RLBCD	right lower border of cardiac dullness
RLE	right lower extremity
RLF	retrolental fibroplasia
RLF	right lateral flexion (back or neck motion)
RLL	right lower lateral
RLL	right lower lobe (lung)
RLLE	right lower lid, eye
RLLLNR	right lower lobe lung, no rales
RLM	right lower medial
RLQ	right lower quadrant (abdomen)
RLR muscle	right lateral rectus muscle
RLS person	person who stammers and cannot enunciate R, L or S
RLSB	right lower scapular border
RLX	right lower extremity
RM	respiratory metabolism
RM	respiratory movement
RMA	Registered Medical Assistant (male nurse)
RMA	right mentoanterior (fetal position)
RMCA	right middle cerebral artery
RMCAT	right middle cerebral artery thrombosis
RMCL	right midclavicular line

RMD	retromanubrial dullness
R-meter	radiation meter
RMF	right middle finger
RML	right mediolateral (episiotomy)
RML	right middle lobe (lung)
RML scar W/O H	right midline scar without hernia
RMP	Regional Medical Program Seminars, financed by Federal Grants for teaching of care of heart disease, cancer, stroke and related diseases Example: CCU course
RMP	right mentoposterior (fetal position)
RMR	right medial rectus (eye muscle)
RMS	root mean square
RMT	right mentotransverse (fetal position)
RN	reactive nitrogen
RN	red nucleus, red nuclei
RN	Registered Nurse
RN	residual nitrogen
Rn	radon
RNA	ribonucleic acid
RNA	rough, non-capsulated, avirulent
RNase	ribonuclease
RNP	ribonucleoprotein
Rnt	roentgenologist, roentgenology
RO, R/O	rule out Example: R/O DU − rule out duodenal ulcer
RO	ratio of

RO	routine order
ROA	right occipitoanterior (fetal position)
R-5-P	ribose- 5- phosphate
ROC	Resident on Call
Roent, roent	roentgenologist, roentgenology
Roent, roent	roentgen ray (xray)
ROM	range of motion
ROM	right otitis media
Rom	Romberg's sign
↓ROM	decreased range of motion
ROM C P	range of motion complete and painfree
ROMSA	right otitis media, suppurative, acute
ROMSCh	right otitis media, suppurative, chronic
ROM WNL	range of motion within normal limits
ROP	right occiput posterior (fetal position)
Ror	Rorschach test
ROS	review of symptoms
ROS	review of systems
ROSS	review of subjective symptoms
ROT	remedial occupational therapy
ROT	right occiput transverse (fetal position)
rot	rotate, rotated, rotation, rotating
rot ny, rot nystag	rotatory nystagmus
rotoscol	rotoscoliosis
ROWTHT	ratio of weight to height

RP	radial pulse
RP	retroperitoneal
RPA	right pulmonary artery
RPCF	Reiter protein complement fixation (test for syphilis)
RPF	relaxed pelvic floor
RPF	renal plasma flow
RPG, rpg	radiation protection guide
R Ph	Registered Pharmacist
RPM	right posterior measurement
rpm	revolutions per minute
RPO	right posterior oblique
RPP	retropubic prostatectomy
RPR test	rapid plasma reagent test
RPS	renal pressor substance
rpt	repeat
rpt	report
RPT	Registered Physical Therapist
rptd	repeated
rptd	reported
RQ	reading quotient
RQ	recovery quotient
RQ	respiratory quotient
RR	radial rate (pulse at wrist)
RR	radiation response

RR	reacting record (electroencephalogram)
RR	Recovery Room
RR	regular rate (heart examination)
RR	respiratory rate
RR	restroom
RR	right rotation (back and neck motion)
RR	Riva-Rocci (sphygmomanometer)
RR cells	radiation reaction cells
R/R	respiratory rate
(no)R or R	no rales or rhonchi (lung examination)
R ₡ R	rate and rhythm (heart examination)
RRAM	rapid alternating movements
RRCT,no(m)	regular rate, clear tones, no murmurs (heart examination)
RRE, RR ₡ E	round, regular and equal (pupils)
RRf	right ring finger
RRL	Registered Record Librarian
RRP	relative refractory period
RRR, RR ₡ R	regular rate and rhythm (heart)
RR=VR	radial rate equals ventricular rate
RS	reinforcing stimulus (psychiatry)
RS	respiratory system
RS	resting subject (not basal, not postabsorptive)
RS	review of symptoms
RS	review of systems

RS ratio	response stimulus ratio
RSA	relative specific activity
RSA	right sacroanterior (fetal position)
RSA → SA	right sacroanterior to sacroanterior
R ScA	right scapuloanterior (fetal position)
RScP	right scapuloposterior (fetal position)
RSO	right salpingo-oophorectomy
RSO	right superior oblique (muscle)
RSP	right sacro posterior (fetal position)
RSR	regular sinus rhythm
RSR s̊ (m)	regular sinus rhythm without murmur
RSS encephalitis	Russian spring-summer encephalitis
RST	right sacrotransverse (fetal position)
RSVC	right superior vena cava
rsvd	reserved
RT	radiation therapy
RT	radiology technician
RT	radium therapy
RT	reaction time
RT	reading test
RT	recreational therapist, recreational therapy
RT	Registered Technician
RT	return to
rt	right
RTC	return to clinic

rt ↓ ext	right lower extremity
rt ↑ ext	right upper extremity
RTF	respiratory tract fluid
rtg, rtgn	roentgen
rtn	return
RTO	return to office
rt ↑ OQ	right upper outer quadrant (buttocks — site of injections)
RTR	Recreational Therapist Registered
rt scap bord	right scapular border
R test	reductase test
RTW	return to work
RU	rat unit
RU	reading unknown
RU	residual urine
RU	retroverted uterus
RU, R unit	Roentgen unit
RU	routine urinalysis
Ru	ruthenium
RUE	right upper extremities, right upper extremity
RUL	right upper lateral
RUL	right upper lobe
RUM	right upper medial
R unit	Roentgen unit
RUOQ	right upper outer quadrant (buttocks)

RUQ	right upper quadrant (abdomen)
rupt	rupture, ruptured
rupt'd	ruptured
rupt memb	ruptured membrane (obstetrics)
RUSB	right upper scapular border
RUX	right upper extremity
RV	rectovaginal
RV	residual volume
RV	retroversion
RV	right ventricle
RV fist	rectovaginal fistula
RVF	renovascular failure
RVH	right ventricular hypertrophy
RVO	relaxed vaginal outlet
RV/TLC	residual volume/ total lung capacity
RW, R/W	return to work
Rx, ℞ *recipe*	any medication or treatment ordered
Rxd, ℞'d	treated
Rx'd US, diath, trx	treated with ultra sound, diathermy, traction
rxn	reaction
rxns	reactions
Rx Phys	treating physician

S	sacral, sacrum
S	scruple (apothecaries weight of 20 grains or one third of a dram)
S	second
S	sedimentation coefficient
S	sensation
S	sensitive
S	serving
S	see
S *semis*	half
S	series
S	sick
S *signa*	label, mark, write, give the following directions (prescription)
S	sign, signed, signature
S *sinestra, sinester*	left
S	single
S	singular
S	sinus
S	sister
S	smooth (bacterial colonies)
S	soft (abdomen, muscle bodies, etc)
S	soft (diet)
S	son
S	space

S
T

S	spherical (lens)
S	stimulus
S	subject
S	sulfur
S	supravergence
S	surgeon, surgical
S	symmetrical
s	second
s	see
s	series
s	singular
s	sinus
s	sister
s	son
s	symmetrical
$\bar{s},\bar{\tilde{s}},\dot{s},\check{s}$, *sine*	without
/S/, /s/	signature, signed Example: /s/ P. Buckley, M.D.
S_1, S_2 etc	sacral nerves or vertebrae by number
S_1, S_2	first heart sound, second heart sound
S_1, S_2, S_3, S_4	suicide risk
SA	scalenus anticus
SA	short arm (cast)
SA	spanish american
SA	surface area (as in area burned, etc.)

SA	sustained action (drug)
S/A	same as above
S/A	short arm (cast)
S-A	sino-atrial, sino-auricular
S ₵ A	sugar and acetone
sa	samarium
sa *secundum artem*	according to the art (using specialized skill)
SAC	short arm cast
sac	sacral, sacrum
sacc	cog wheel (respiration)
sacc	short arm cylinder cast
sacch	saccharine
SACH	solid ankle, cushion heel
sac-il	sacro-iliac
SAD (test)	sugar, acetone, diacetic acid test
SAE	short above elbow
SAH	subarachnoid hemorrhage
Sal	salmonella
sal *secundum artes leges*	according to the rules of the art (pharmacy)
san, sanit	sanitarium
sanit	sanitary, sanitation
SAP	serum acid phospate
sap, sapon, saponif	saponification, saponify
Sar	sulpharphenamine

SAT	Scholastic Aptitude Test
SAT (chromosone)	chromosone with satellite
SAT *sino acido thymonucleinico*	without thymonucleic acid
sat	satisfactory
sat	saturate, saturated
sat cond	satisfactory condition
sat'd	saturated
satis, satisf	satisfactory
satn	saturation
sat sol	saturated solution
sat sol KI	saturated solution of potassium iodine (Lugol's solution)
SB	sandbag
SB	Bachelor of Science
SB	southbound (description of position of vehicle in accident)
SB (test)	Stanford-Binet test
SB	stillborn
Sb *stibium*	antimony
Sb	strabismus
SBD	senile brain disease
SBE	short below elbow
SBE	subacute bacterial endocarditis
SBO	small bowel obstruction
SBR	strict bed rest

S by S	symptoms by systems
SC	closure of semilunar valves
SC	schedule change
SC	self care
SC	service connected (injury or illness incurred in line of duty in military service — occasionally used in reference to civilian occupations)
SC	sickle cell disease
SC	conditioned stimulus
SC	subcutaneous
Sc	scandium
Sc	scapula, scapular
Sc, sc	conditioned stimulus
sc	scant
sc	scapula
sc	science, scientific
sc *scilicet*	namely; it is permitted to know
sc	sclera
$\dot{s}$ c	without correction
½ Sc	medioregiones infraspinatus scapulae
S $\not{c}$ C	singly and consensually (eyes)
SCA	School and College Ability (Tests)
scap	scapula, scapular
SCAT, SCA tests	School and College Ability Tests
SCAT	sheep cell agglutination test

SCB	sedative cabinet bath
SCB	strictly confined to bed
SCD	Service Connected Disability (military, civil or industrial)
SCD, SC disease	sickle cell disease
SCD	surgeon's certificate of disability
ScD	Doctor of Science
Sc DA *scapula dextra anterior*	scapular right anterior (fetal position)
Sc DP *scapula dextra posterior*	scapular right posterior (fetal position)
scf/min	standard cubic feet per minute
sched	schedule, scheduled
SCI	spinal cord injury
sci	science, scientific
scint	scintogram
Scl, scl	sclerosis, sclerotic
ScLA *scapula laeva anterior*	left scapuloanterior (fetal position)
ScLP *scapula laeva posterior*	left scapuloposterior (fetal position)
SCM	Schwann cell membrane
SCM	sensation, circulation and motion (notes made when checking fingers or toes of an injured extremity)
SCM	sternocleidomastoid (muscle)
SCM	surface connecting membrane
SC & M	sensation, circulation and motion (fingers or toes of injured extremity)

scop	scopolamine
SCR	Schick Conversion rate
scr	scruple
SCRAP	Simplex Complex Reaction Time Apparatus
Scripts, scripts	prescriptions
scrup	scruple
sc sp	scapular spine
SCU	Special Care Unit
SCUBA	self-contained underwater breathing apparatus
SCV	smooth, capsulated, virulent
SD	scotch douche
SD	shoulder disarticulation
SD	standard deviation
SD	stimulus drive
SD	streptodornase
S-D	strength-duration (curve)
SDA *sacro dextro anterior*	right sacral anterior (fetal position)
SDA	specific dynamic action
SDA	succinus dehydrogenase activity
SDH	succinic dehydrogenase
sdly	sidelying
SDM	single, divorced, married
SDP *sacro dextro posterior*	right sacral posterior (fetal position)
sds	sounds

SDT   right sacral transverse (fetal position)
   sacro dextra tranversa

SDU   short double upright (brace)

SDUB   short double upright brace

SE   saline enema

SE   spherical equivalent

SE   standard error

Se   selenium

S ¢ E   skeletal and extremities (physical examination)

SEA (test)   sheep erythrocyte agglutination test

SEA   spontaneous electrical activity (physiology)

SEC   soft elastic capsule

Sec   seconal

sec   secant

sec   second (unit of time)

sec   second, secondary (numerical order)

sec   section, sectioned, sectioned

sech   hyperbolic secant

sect   section, sectioned, sections

secy   secretary

SED   suberythemal dose

Sed (rate, test, time)   sedimentation

sed   sedate, sedated

sed   sedimentation

sed   stool
   sedes

SEE	Scopolamine-Eakodal-Ephetonin
seg, segm	segment, segmented
segs	segmented neutrophils (hematology)
sem	semen, seminal
sem *semis*	half
semidr *semidrachma*	half a dram
semih *semihora*	half hour
sem ves	seminal vesicle
sen	sensation
↓ sen	diminished sensation
sens	senses, sensation, sensitive, sensorium, sensory
↓ sens	decreased sensation, diminished sensation
sens decr	sensation decreased
sens defic	sensory deficit
sens lat *sensu lato*	in the broad sense
sens str *sensu stricto*	in the strict sense
sep	separate, separated, separation
sept	septum
sept *septem*	seven
seq *sequela*	that which follows
seq	sequence

seq, seqq *sequentiae*	the following
seq luce *sequenti luce*	the following day
Ser	serology
ser	serial, serially, series
ser	serological, serology
ser	serous
ser	serum
ser cl	serum chloride
ser ind	serum index
serol	serology
serosang	serosanguinous
ser sect	serial section
serv *serva*	service, services
serv	keep, preserve
sesquih *sesquihora*	an hour and a half
sev	sever, severed
sev	several
sev	severe
SF	salt free (diet)
SF	scarlet fever
SF	spinal fluid
Sf, S_f	Svedberg flotation units
SFC	spinal fluid count

SF def	silver fork deformity (fracture of wrist)
SFF	speaking fundamental frequency
s fr *spiritus frumenti*	whiskey
SFU	surgical follow up
SG	specific gravity
SG	Surgeon General
Sg, sg	specific gravity
sg	sign (objective finding)
S-G (test)	Sachs-Georgi test
s-g	subgenus
s-gg	subgenera
sgs	signs (objective findings)
SGO	Surgeon General's Office
SGOT	serum glutamic oxaloacetic transaminase
SGPT	serum glutamic pyruvic transaminase
SH	self help
SH	percentage saturation of hemoglobin
SH	serum hepatitis
SH	social history
SH	somatotropic (growth) hormone
SH	State Hospital
Sh	shigella
Sh	short
Sh	shoulder

sh	short
sh	shoulder
SHF	super high frequency
Shig	shigella (bacteriology)
shl, shld, shldr	shoulder
S hormone	"sugar" hormone (Fuller Albright) glycogenic corticoids
sho, should	shoulder
SHS	Sayre head sling
SI	sacroiliac
SI	saturation index
SI	seriously ill
SI	soluble insulin
SI	stress incontinence
Si	silicon
SI jt	sacroiliac joint
SI list	seriously ill list
SI units	International System of units
sib	sibling
sibs	siblings
sic (not an abbreviation)	so
sicc *siccus*	dry
SID *semel in die*	once a day
Sif	segment inferior (gynecology)

SIG	sigmoidoscope, sigmoidoscopic, sigmoidoscopy
Sig, sig *signa*	label, write, give the following directions (prescription)
Sig	signature, signed
sig F	significant findings
sig n pro *signa nomine proprio*	label with proper name (pharmacy)
SIJ	sacroiliac joint
SIL	sister-in-law
Sim, simul	simultaneous
sin	sinus
sine (not an abbreviation)	without
sing	single
sing	singular
Sinh, Sin h	hyperbolic sine
sis	sister
si non val *si non valeat*	if it is not enough
SIT	supraspinatus, infraspinatus, teres minor (muscle group)
sitg	sitting
si vir perm *si vires permitant*	if strength permits
SK	streptokinase
sk	skeletal
sk	skimmed
skel	skeletal

sk tr, sk trx, sk tx	skeletal traction
SL	Serious List
SL	short leg (cast)
SL	small leucocyte
sl	slice
sl	slight, slightly
s l, s lat *sensu lato*	in the broad sense
SLA *sacro laeva anterior*	sacrum left anterior (fetal position)
SLB	short leg brace
sl blad inf	slight bladder infection
sl bt	slightly better
SLC	short leg cast
SLCC	short leg cylinder cast
SLD	serum lactic acid dehydrogenase
SLE	slit lamp examination (ophthalmology)
SLE	St. Louis encephalitis
SLE	systemic lupus erythematosus
SLP *sacro laeva posterior*	left sacroposterior (fetal position)
SLP of P cast	short leg plaster of paris cast
SLR	straight leg raising
SLT *sacro laeva transversa*	left sacrum transversa (fetal position)
slt	slight, slightly
sl tr	slight trace

SLW	short leg walking (cast or boot)
SLWC	short leg walking cast
SM	streptomycin
SM	systolic murmur
Sm	samarium
sm	small
SMA	superior mesentery artery
SMA	Trade name for a baby formula which stands for "synthetic mild adapted"
SMD	senile macular degeneration (eyes)
SMD	submanubrial dullness
SMDSep	single, married, divorced, separated (indication of marital status on insurance papers, admitting records, etc.)
SMO	Senior Medical Officer
SMPS	sulfated mucopolysaccharides
SMR	submucous resection
SN	scrub nurse (operating room)
SN	spinal needle (usually written with length and gauge size — Example: SN#20 2½″)
SN	student nurse
SN *stannum*	tin
sn *secundum naturam*	according to nature
S/N ratio	speech to noise ratio
SNAFU	situation normal, all fouled up
SNB	scalene node biopsy

SNB	Silverman needle biopsy
SNC *sistema nervoso centrale*	central nervous system
SNDO	Standard Nomenclature of Diseases and Operations
SNM	Society of Nuclear Medicine
SNS	sympathetic nervous system
SNST	sciatic nerve stretch test
SNT	sinuses, nose and throat
SO	salpingo-oophorectomy
SO	supraorbital
SO	sutures out
S-O, S ⊄ O	salpingo-oophorectomy
SO$_4$	sulfate
SOA	symptoms of asthma
SOAM, SO/a.m.	sutures out in a.m.
SOB	see order book
SOB	shortness of breath
SOB	suboccipitobregmatic
soc	social, society
Soc Sec	social security
Soc Serv	social service
Soc Hist	social history
sod	soda, sodium
soda bicarb, sod bicarb	sodium bicarbonate
Sod Pent	sodium pentothal (anesthetic)

SOER	special orthopedic examination and report
S of B	shortness of breath
SOFT	Sorting of Figures Test
Sol	solarium (in some hospitals, the ward name)
sol	soluble
sol	solution
solidif	solidification
soln	solution
Solu B c̄ C	solution of soluble B vitamins with vitamin C (trade name)
Solut, solut	solution
solv	solvent
som, somat	somatic
SON	supraoptic nuclei
SONP	soft organs not palpable
SOP	standard operating procedure
SOPM, SO/p.m.	sutures out in p.m.
s op s *si opus sit*	if necessary
S-O-R	stimulus-organism-response
SOS *si opus sit*	if necessary (used to indicate that an order may be given *once only if necessary* whereas prn orders may be given at stated intervals whenever necessary)
SOS	stimulation of senses
SOTT	synthetic medium old tuberculin
SP	semiprivate

Sp	spirometer
sp	sacropubic, sacrum to pubis
sp	space
sp	spasm
sp	species (singular)
sp	specific
sp	spine, spinal
sp	splint
sp	spiritus (pharmacy)
S-P (nail)	Smith-Peterson nail
S/P	status post Example: S/P craniotomy sat = status post craniotomy satisfactory
sp an	spinal anesthesia
spans	spansule (timed delayed action capsule)
SPCA	serum prothrombin conversion accelerator
SPCC	Society for Prevention of Cruelty to Children
sp cd	spinal cord
SPD	sociopathic personality disorder
spec	special
spec	specific
spec	specification
spec	specimen
specif	specific, specification, specified
sp fl	spinal fluid
spg, sp gr	specific gravity

sph	spherical (lens)
sph	sphincter
S phen	Smith's phenomenon
sp ht	specific heat
SPI	serum precipitable iodine
SPI	serum protein index
sp indet	species indeterminate
sp inquir *species inquirendae*	species of doubtful status
spir	spiral
spir	spiritual
spir	spiritus (pharmacy)
spir	spirochaeta (pathology)
spl	splint
SPM	Syndrome Pierre Mauriac (obesity and hepatomegaly and retarded growth associated with diabetes mellitus)
sp mening	spinal meningitis
SPN	student practical nurse
SP nail	Smith-Peterson nail
spn, sp nov *species novum*	new species
Sp Ny	spontaneous nystagmus
sp o.k.	speech o.k.
spon, spnt	spontaneous
SPP	superior patellar pole
SPP	suprapubic prostatectomy

spp	species (plural)
sp pr, sp proc	spinal process
SPPS	stable plasma protein solution
spr	sprain
spt	spirit (pharmacy)
spiritus	
SP tube	suprapubic tube
Spur	Spurling test
sp xr	special xray study
SPZ	sulfipyrazone
SQ	status quo
SQ	subcutaneous, subcutaneously
sq	the following
sequentia	
sq	square
sq cell ca	sqamous cell carcinoma
sq cm	square centimeter
sq ft	square foot
sq in	square inch
sq m	square meter
sq mm	square millimeter
sqq	the following
sequentiae	
SQ_3R	survey, question, read, review, recite
SR	schizophrenic reaction
SR	sedimentation rate

SR (cells)	sensitization response cells
SR	shortening range
SR	sinus rhythm
SR	stimulus response
SR	stomach rumble
SR	stretch reflex
SR	supply room
SR	system review
S/R	schizophrenic reaction
Sr	senior
Sr	sigma reaction
Sr	strontium
sr	steradian
SR ac undiff	schizophrenic reaction, acute, undifferentiated
SR/AP	schizophrenic reaction, acute, paranoid
SR/AU	schizophrenic reaction, acute, undifferentiated
SR/CP	schizophrenic reaction, chronic, paranoid
SR/CU	schizophrenic reaction, chronic, undifferentiated
Srg, srg	surgery
SRS	slow reacting substance
SS	saline soak
SS	sitting, standing
SS	skull series (xrays)
SS	soap solution
SS	soap suds

SS   social service

SS   special senses

SS   special services

SS   standard score

SS   sterile solution

SS   suction socket

SS   surging sine

S/S (diet)   salt substitute diet

ss   sacrosciatic

s̄s̄, s̄s̄, śś, ss   one half
  semis

ss   in the strict sense
  sensu stricto

ss   subjects

ss   symptoms

S ₡ S   signs and symptoms

S or S   signs or symptoms

SSA   special somatic afferent

SS agar   Shigella and Salmonella agar

SSB   Social Security Benefits

SSCQT   Selective Service College Qualifying Test

SSD   source to skin distance

SSE   soap solution enema, soap suds enema

s̄ seq   without sequela

SSIT   subscapularis, supraspinatus, infraspinatus, teres
                               minor (muscle group)

SSKI	saturated solution of potassium iodine
SSMGSO$_4$	saturated solution of magnesium sulfate
SSMS	saturated solution of magnesium sulfate
ss notch	sacro-sciatic notch
SSS	special soluble substance
SSS	sterile saline soak
sss *stratum supra stratum*	layer upon layer
s str *sensu stricto*	in the strict sense
SSU	Saybolt seconds universal
SSU	self service unit
SS $\cancel{c}$ US	surging sine and ultra sound
SSV, ssv *sub signo veneni*	under a poison label
ST	sedimentation time
ST	shock therapy
ST	slight trace
ST	speech therapy
ST	standardized test
ST	surface tension
ST	survival time
st	standing
st	status
st *stet*	let it stand
st	stimulus, stimuli, stimulation

st	stone
st	straight
st	strength
st	stretch
St_{37}	hexylresorcinol
↓ST	depressed ST segment (electocardiogram)
ST (platform)	sustentaculum tali platform (orthopedics)
ST (segment)	part of electrocardiogram pattern
sta	station
St AE	standard above elbow
stan, stand	standard, standarized, standardization
staph	staphylococcal, staphylococcus
Stap mob, Stapes mob	stapes mobilization
STAT, Stat *statim*	at once, immediately
stat, statist	statistics, statisical
stb	stillborn
STC	somatotropin, corticosterone, 1-thyroxine
STD	skin test dose
STD	standard test dose
std	stand
std	standard, standardized, standardization
stdg	standing
ster	sterile
stereo	stereogram

stern punct	sternal puncture
STH	somatotrophic hormone (growth hormone)
stillat *stillatim*	by drops or in small quantities
stim, stimul	stimulate, stimulation, stimulus
STL	swelling, tenderness and limitation
STLOM	swelling, tenderness and limitation of motion
stom	stomach
stom lav → cl	stomach gavage (tube feeding)
stom lav	stomach lavage (washing out of stomach contents)
stom lav→cl	stomach lavage to clear
STP	standard temperature and pressure
STPD	standard temperature and pressure, dry
ST platform	sustentaculum tali platform (orthopedics)
St pr *status praesens*	present status
STPS	standard temperature and pressure, saturated
STR	soft tissue relaxation
Str	streptococcus
str	straight
str	strain, strained
str	strength
str	streptococcus
str	stretch
str	strong (heart sounds)

strab	strabismus
Strep, strep, strept, streptoc	streptococcus
struct	structure, structural
STS	serological test for syphilis
ST seg	ST segment (electrocardiogram)
STSG	split thickness skin graft (plastic surgery)
sttg	sitting
STU	skin test unit
STVB	Strong Vocational Interest Blank
SU	secretory units
SU	sensation unit (psychiatry or neurology)
SU	sigma units (as in alkaline phosphatase)
su	subject
su *sumat*	let him take
su	surgeon, surgical, surgery
sub	substitute
subac	subacute
subclav	subclavian, subclavicular
subclin	subclinical
subcr, subcrep	subcrepitant
subcu, subcut	subcutaneous, subcutaneously
sub fin coct *sub finem coctionis*	toward the end of boiling
subgen	subgenus
subj	subject, subjective

subj sx	subjective symptoms
subl	sublime, sublimate, sublimation
subl, subling	sublingual, sublingually
sublux	subluxation
submand	submandibular
suboccip	suboccipital
suborb stim	suborbital stimulation
suboccip	suboccipital
subq, sub-q	subcutaneous
subsc, subscap	subscapular
subsp	subspecies
subst	substance
subst	substitute
substd	substandard
SUD	skin unit dose
SUD syndrome	sudden unexpected death syndrome
SUDI	sudden unexpected death of infant
suf, suff	sufficient
sug	sugar
sug	suggest
sulf	sulfate
SUHT	subject's height in inches
sum *sumati*	let it be taken
sum *sumendum*	let them be taken

sum tal   take one each
  sumati tales

sup   superficial

sup   superior

sup   supination

sup   supine

sup   above
  supra

superf, superfic   superficial

superimp   superimpose, superimposed

supp   suppository

supp   suppurative

sup pat (pole)   superior patellar pole

suppl   supplement, supplemental

suppos   suppository

supra (not an abbreviation)   superior, above

supra cit   cited above
  supra citato

supra pat   supra patellar

supt   superintendent

supv   supervisor, supervision

surg   surgeon, surgery, surgical

surgs   surgeons

susc   susceptible, susceptible, susceptibility

susp   suspension

sut   suture

SV	simian virus
SV	sinus venosus
SV	stroke volume
sv	single vibrations
sv *spiritus vini*	alcoholic spirits
SVA	special visceral afferent
SVC	superior vena cava
SVE	special visceral efferent
svg *spiritus vini gallici*	brandy
SVIB	Strong Vocational Interest Blank
SVR, svr *spiritus vini rectificatus*	alcohol
$S_1 VR$, $S_2 VR$	sacral ventral root by number
svt *spiritus vini tenius*	proof spirit
SW	short wave
SW	sine wave
SW	stab wound
sw	sweet
sw	swelling
SWD	sine wave diathermy
SW dia, SW diath	short wave diathermy, sine wave diathermy
SWR	serum Wasserman reaction
sx	signs (if listed as findings)
sx	symptoms (if listed as complaints)

sx↑	symptoms increased
sx↓	symptoms decreased
sx & sx	signs and symptoms
sym	symptom
sym .	symmetrical, symmetry
symb	symbol, symbolic
symp	sympathetic
symp	symptom
sympath	sympathetic
symp sys	sympathetic system
syn	synergist, synergy
syn	synonym
syn	synovial
synd	syndrome
synov	synovial, synovitis, synovectomy
syph	syphilis, syphilitic
sys	system
sys	systolic
sys m	systolic murmur
syst	system
syst	systolic

T	tablespoon
T	temperature
T	temporal (skull area)
T	tender, tenderness
T	tension (intraocular)
T _tera_	monster
T _tesla_	high frequency oscillating current of medium voltage used in electrotherapy
T	therapist
T	thoracic
T	time, timing
T	tincture
T	tone
T	topical
T	total
T	trace
T	transition point
T	transverse
T	treponema
T	tritium
T	tuberculin, tuberculosis, tuberculous
T wave	a part of the electrocardiogram pattern
T/	than
T/	then
T/	transfers

t	teaspoon
t	temperature
t	time
T_1, T_2, T_3 or T1, T2, T3 etc	thoracic nerves or thoracic vertebrae by number
T+1, T+2, T+3	stages of increased intraocular pressure
T−1, T−2, T−3	stages of decreased intraocular pressure
T_3	triiodothyronine uptake
T↓	tension decreased (intraocular)
T↑	tension increased (intraocular)
T↓↓	testicles both descended
T↑	tourniquet (pneumatic) inflated
T↓	tourniquet (pneumatic) released
TA	temperature axillary
TA	Tendon of Achilles
TA	tension, arterial
TA	toxin antitoxin
TA	traffic accident
TA	transaldolase
TA	tryptophane acid (reaction)
TA	tuberculin alkaline
T ȼ A	tonsils and adenoids, tonsillectomy and adenoid-ectomy, tonsillitis and adenoiditis
Ta	tantalum
TAB	typhoid, paratyphoid A and paratyphoid B (vaccine)
tab	tablet

TACE	trianisylchloroethylene
tach, tachy	tachycardia
TAF *Tuberculin Albumose Frei*	albumin free tuberculin
TAF	toxoid, antitoxin floccules
TAH	total abdominal hysterectomy
tal *talis*	such a one
TAM	toxoid, antitoxin mixture
TAME	tosylarginine methylester
tan	tangent
tanh	hyperbolic tangent
TAO	thromboangiitis obliterans (Buerger's disease)
TAO	triacetyloleandomycin
TAT	Tell a Tale (psychiatry)
TAT	tetanus antitoxin
TAT	Thematic Apperception Test
TAT	toxin antitoxin
TATBA	triamcinolone acetonide tertiary butyl acetate
TATST	tetanus antitoxin skin test
TB	thymol blue
TB	total body
Tb	terbium
Tb, tb	tuberculosis
TBA	tertiary butyl acetate
TBA	thiobarbituric acid

TBA	thyroxin binding albumin
TBB 1-698	tibione (tuberculostatic medication)
Tbc, tbc	tubercle bacillus, tuberculosis
tbcn	tuberculin
TBE	tuberculin bacillen emulsion
TBG	thyroxin binding globulin
TBLC	term birth, living child
TBLI	term birth, living infant
TBP	thyroxin binding protein
TBPA	thyroxin binding prealbumin
tbs, tbsp	tablespoon
TBW, TBWA	total body water
TC	telephone call
TC	teracycline
TC	tissue culture
TC	to contain
TC	tuberculin, contagious
T/C	telephone call
Tc	technetium
Tc, tc	telephone call
T ¢ C	turn and cough
T ¢ C	type and crossmatch
TCA	trichloracetic acid
TCC	thromboplastic cell component
TCE	tetrachlorodiphenylethane

TCD, TCD₀₀	tissue culture dose
TCP	tricresyl phosphate
T ¢ CrM	type and cross match
TD	terminal device
TD	typhoid dysentery
TDE	tetrachlorodiphenylethane
TDN	totally digestible nutrients
TDS *ter die sumendum*	take three times a day
TE	tonsils excised
TE, T ¢ E	trial and error
Te	tellurium
TEA	thromboendarterectomy
TEAB	tetraethylammonium bromide
TEAC	tetraethylammonium chloride
tech	technic, technical, technician
techn	technician
TED	threshold erythema dose (radiology)
TEF, TE fist	tracheoesophageal fistula
TEM	triethylene melamine
temp	temperature
temp	temple
temp	temporal (refers to temple)
temp	temporary
temp dext *temperi dextro*	to the right temple

temp sinist *temperi sinistro*	to the left temple
ten	tense, tension
tend	tender, tenderness
tens	tension
tent	tentative
tent diag	tentative diagnosis
TEPA	triethylenephosphoramide
TEPP	tetraethylpyrophosphate
ter *tere*	rub
term	terminal
term	termination
tert	tertiary
tertipara, para III	third pregnancy (to viable period)
tet	tetanus, tetany
TETRAC	tetraiodothyroacetic acid
TF	tactile fremitus
TF	to follow
TF	tuning fork
TF	tuberculin filtrate
tf	to follow
tf	tuning fork
T of F	tetrology of Fallot
tg	type genus
TGE	transmissable gastroenteritis

TGE agar	tryptone glucose extract milk agar
TGT	thromboplastin generation test
TH	thyroid hormone
Th	thoracic, thorax
Th	thorium
Th	thoron
Th	thyroid
THC	delta 1 tetrahydrocanabinol (a chemical present in marijuana which causes the hallucinations, etc.)
ther	therapeutic, therapy
therm	thermolite (metal reinforced porcelain used for dental crowns)
therm	thermometer
th ex	therapeutic exercises
THC	tetrahydrocortisone
THF	tetrahydro F
THFA	tetrahydrofuryl alcohol
THI, Thi	thiamin
Thor, thor	thoracic, thorax
THR	threonine
thr	thrill
throm, thromb	thrombosis, thrombus
TI	tricuspid insufficiency (heart)
TI	transverse diameter between ischia (pelvic measurement)
Ti	titanium

TIA	transient ischemia attacks
tib	tibia
tib plat	tibial plateau
tic	particularly
TID, tid *ter in die*	three times a day
TIN, tin *ter in nocte*	three times during the night
tinct	tincture
ting	tingling
T in ml	tongue in midline (neurology)
TIW, tiw	three times in a week
TJ	triceps jerk (deep tendon reflex)
TK	transketolase
TKA	trochanter, knee, ankle alignment
TKD	tokodynamometer
TKG	tokodynagraph
TL	terminal limen
TL	total lung capacity
TL	tubal ligation
Tl	thallium
TLC	tender loving care (written on children's and aged person's charts to indicate that the patient should have emotional support)
TLC	total lung capacity
TLR	tonic labyrinthine reflex
TM	temperature by mouth

TM	temporomandibular
TM	tender midline
TM	tympanic membrane
TM	maximal tubular excretory capacity (kidney)
tm	true mean
T ₵ M, T ₵ xM	type and cross match (blood)
TmG, Tm (g)	maximum tubular reabsorption rate for glucose
TMJ, TM jt	temporomandibular joint
TML, T/ML	tender midline
TML	tongue in midline
Tm PAH	maximum tubular excretory capacity for PAH
TMTD	tetramethylthiuramdisulphide
TMT, T-MT	tarsometatarsal
Tmt, tmt	treatment
TMV	tobacco mosaic virus
TN	tarsonavicular
Tn	normal intraocular tension
Tn	thoron
TNC	too numerous to count (laboratory)
TNR	tonic neck reflex
tns	tension
tnsn	tension
TNTC	too numerous to count
TO	target organ
TO	telephone order

TO	transfer out (as from Intensive Care Unit to the ward or from the hospital to a convalescent home, etc.)
TO	temperature, oral
TO	thrown off (horse, bicycle, motorcycle, etc)
TO	thrown out (of car in accident)
TO *tintua opii*	tincture of opium
TO	trachelotomy and oophorectomy
TO	tuberculin old
TO	tuberculin original
T-O	trachelotomy and oophorectomy
TOA	tubo-ovarian abscess
T of F	tetrology of Fallot
tol	tolerance, tolerated
tonoc	tonight
top	topical
tot	total
tow	to other ward
TOWER	Testing, Orientation and Work Evaluation for Rehabilitation
tox	toxic, toxicity, toxin, toxology
TP	temporoparietal
TP	tissue pressure
TP	toilet paper
TP	total protein
TP	transverse process

TP	treponema pallidum
TP	tuberculin precipitation
TP *tuberculosis pulmonum*	pulmonary tuberculosis
T-P	temporoparietal
T ₵ P	temperature and pulse
TPC	thromboplastic plasma component
TPC (test)	treponema pallidum complement test
TPCF	treponema pallidum complement fixation test
TPD	temporary partial disability
TPIA	treponema pallidum immune adherence test
TPI (test)	treponema pallidum immobilization test
TPN	triphosphopyridine nucleotide
TPNH	triphosphopyridine nucleotide, reduced form
TPO	tryptophan peroxidase
TPP	thiamine pyrophosphate
TPR	temperature, pulse and respiration
TPR	total peripheral resistance
TPT	tetraphenyl tetrazolium
TPT	total protein tuberculin
TR, T/R	temperature rectal
TR	therapeutic radiology (special field of radiology)
TR	tuberculin R
TR	turbidity reducing
Tr	terbium

Tr	tincture
Tr	transfer
tr	tincture
tr	trace
tr	traction
tr	transfer
tr	trauma
tr	treatment
tr	tremor
T ∉ R	tenderness ∉ rebound
T or R	tenderness or rebound
trach	trachea
trach	tracheostomy, tracheotomy
trach	trachoma
trans	transaction
trans	transfer, transferred
trans	transilluminate (sinuses)
trans	transverse
transm	transmission
transpl	transplant
trans sect	transverse section
transv proc	transverse process (vertebra)
transv sect	transverse section
trap	trapezius

trem, tremb	trembling
Trend	Trendelenberg (position)
trep	treponema (bacteriology)
trg	training
TRI	Total Response Index (psychiatry)
tri	triceps
Trich, trich	trichomonas
trid *tridium*	three days
trig	trigger
trig	trigonal
trig pnt, trig pt	trigger point
tr ₵ imp	treated and improved
TRIT	trithyronine
trit	triturate
TRO	to return to office
troch	trochanter
troch *trochiscus*	lozenge
Trop Med	Tropical Medicine (designation of medical specialty)
TRP	Tactical Reproduction Pegboard
TRP	tubular reabsorption of phosphate trytophan
trt	treatment
TR unit, Tr unit	turbidity reducing unit
TRX, trx	traction

trx	treatments
TS	tensile strength
TS	terminal sensation
TS	test solution
TS	thoracic surgery
TS	thyroid serum
TS	toe signs
TS	tracheal sound
TS	tricuspid stenosis
TS	triple strength
TS	tubular sound
T state	tension state
TSB	total serum bilirubin
TSD	target skin distance
T sect	transverse section
TSH	thyroid stimulating hormone
TSI agar	triple sugar iron agar
TSP	thyroid stimulating hormone of the anterior pituitary
tsp	teaspoon
TSTA	toxoplasmin skin test antigen
TT	tactile tension
TT	test tube
TT	tetanus toxoid
TT	thymol turbidity

TT	tilt table
TT	transferred to
TT	transit time (of blood through the heart)
(no)T or T	no thrust or thrill (heart)
TTD	temporary total disability
TTD	transverse thoracic diameter
TTH	thyrotropic hormone
TTP	tritolyl phosphate
TTR	triceps tendon reflex
TTS	tilt table standing
TTT	total twitch time
TU	toxic unit
Tu	transmission unit
TUR	transurethral resection
tur	turgor
turb	turbid, turbidity
turb	turbinate
turg	turgor
TURP	transurethral resection, prostate
turp	turpentine
TUS	take up strap
tus *tussis*	cough
TV	tetrazolium violet
TV	tidal volume

TV	Toucher vaginal
TV	total volume
TV	trial visit
TV	trichomonas vaginalis
TV	tuberculin volutin
TV	typhus vaccine
TVC	timed vital capacity
T_2VR, TVr_2	thoracic ventral root nerve by number
TWE, TW enema	tap water enema
TWHW ok	toe walking and heel walking all right
Tx, tx	traction
Tx, tx	treatments
T ₵ C, T ₵ Xmatch	type and crossmatch (blood for transfusion) Example: T & C 2UWB = type and cross match two units whole blood
tymp	tympanic, tympanicity, tympany
tymp memb	tympanic membrane (ear drum)
typ	typical
TZ	tuberculin zymoplastiche

U	ulna, ulnar
U	umbilicus
U	unable (because of physical disability)
U	unit
U	university
U	upper
U	uranium
U	urea
U	urine
U	urology
U	uterus
u	ulna
u	unit
u	urea
U/2	upper half
U/3	upper third
UA (sound)	ultra audible sound
UA	uric acid
UA	urinalysis
ua *usque ad*	up to, as far as
UB, Ub	upper back
UB	urinary bladder
UBA	undenatured bacterial antigen
UBI	ultraviolet blood irradiation

U
V

UC	unconscious
UC	uterine contractions
U ₡ C	urethral and cervical
UCD, UCHD	usual childhood diseases
UCD s̄ seq	usual childhood diseases without sequelae
UCI	usual childhood illnesses
UCL, U Cl	urea clearance test
UCPA	United Cerebral Palsy Association
UCR	unconditioned reflex
UCR	unconditioned response
UCS	unconditioned stimulus
UCV	uncontrolled variable
UD	ulnar deviation
UD	under developed
UD	urethral drainage
UD	uridine diphosphate
UD	urinary drainage
ud *ut dictum*	as directed
UDC	usual diseases of childhood
UDPG	uridine diphosphate glucose
UDPGA	uridine diphosphate glucaronic acid
UE	undetermined etiology
UE	under elbow
UE	upper extremity, upper extremities

U ext, U/ext	upper extremity, upper extremities
UEG	echoencephalogram
UEG	ultrasonic encephalogram
UFR	urine filtration rate
UG	undergraduate nurse
UG	urogenital
UGI	upper gastrointestinal
UHF	ultra high frequency
ULLE	upper lid, left eye
ULQ	upper left quadrant
ULRE	upper lid, right eye
ult	ultimately
ult praes *ultimum praesriptus*	as last prescribed
UM	upper motor neuron
umb	umbilicus, umbilical
umb reg	umbilical region
UMN	upper motor neuron
UMNL	upper motor neuron lesion
U ⊄ M NP	ulnar and median nerve palsy
UMP	uracil monophosphate
un	unable
unacc	unaccompanied
unc	unconscious
uncert	uncertain, uncertainties

unchg	unchanged
uncomp	uncompensated
uncompl	uncomplicated
uncond	unconditioned
uncond ref	unconditioned reflex
uncond resp	unconditioned response
uncoop	uncooperative
uncor	uncorrected
unCS	unconditioned stimulus
undet	undetermined
undet etiol	undetermined etiology
undet orig	undetermined origin
ung *unguentum*	ointment
unilat	unilateral
unipara	a woman who has had one pregnancy which has gone to the period of viability
univ	universal, universally
univ	university
unoff	unofficial
unrem, unremit	unremitting
UnS, un s	unconditioned stimulus
uns	unsaturated
unsat	unsatisfactory
unsat	unsaturated
unst	unstable

unst	unsteady
unsw	unsweetened
unsym	unsymmetrical
UO	undetermined origin
U/O adeq	urine output adequate
UO	urinary output
UO, U/O	under observation
UOQ	upper outer quadrant (buttocks)
U/P	urine/plasma concentration ratios
up ad lib	up (out of bed) as desired
up OOB ad lib	up (out of bed) as desired
UQ	upper quadrant
UR	unconditioned reflex, unconditioned response
UR, Ur	urologist, urology (medical specialty)
Ur	uranium
ur	urine
ur anal	urine analysis
URI	upper respiratory infection
uro-gen	urinogenital
urol	urological, urologist, urology
URQ	upper right quadrant
US	ultra sound
US	unconditioned stimulus
us	as above
ut supra	

USAFMC	United States Air Force Medical Corps
USAMC, USA (MC)	United States Army Medical Corps
USD	United States Dispensatory
USDHEW	United States Department of Health Education and Welfare
USNMC	United States Navy Medical Corps
USP, USPhar	United States Pharmacopoeia
USPHS	United States Public Health Service
USVA	United States Veterans Administration
USVAH	United States Veterans Administration Hospital
USVB	United States Veterans Bureau
USVH	United States Veterans Hospital
ut dict *ut dictum*	as directed
ut supr *ut supra*	as above
utend *utendus*	to be used
UTI	urinary tract infection
UTOC	upper thoracic outlet compression syndrome
UTP	uridine triphosphate
UU	urine urobilin
UV	ultra violet
UVR	ultra violet radiation
U/WB	unit of whole blood
Ux	urinalysis

V	Roman numeral 5
V	valve
V	vanadium
V	unipolar chest lead in electrocardiogram
V	vector
V	velosity
V	venous
V	ventral
V	ventricle, ventricular
V	verbal
V	versus (against)
V	vertex
V	vestibular
V (factor)	verbal comprehension factor
V	vibrio
V *vide*	see
V	view
V	virulence
V	vision, visual
V	volt
V	volume
V #1, V #2	vehicle number one etc. in description of vehicular accident
V_1	ophthalmic division of fifth cranial nerve
V_2	maxillary division of fifth cranial nerve

V_3	mandibular division of fifth cranial nerve
V^+ (substance)	kynurenine
v	valve
v	vein
v	venous
v	ventral
v	ventricle, ventricular
v	verbal
v	versus (against)
v	vertex
v	volt
v	volume
VA	Veterans Administration
VA	visual acuity
VA	anatomical volume
va	volt ampere
vac	vacuum
vacc	vaccine, vaccination
V Ad, Vadj	vocational adjustment
V Adm	Veteran's Administration
vag	vagina, vaginal
VAH	Veteran's Administration Hospital
VAL	valine
VAOD	visual acuity, right eye
VAOS	visual acuity, left eye

VAOU	visual acuity, both eyes
VA↓OD	visual acuity decreased in right eye
VA↓OS	visual acuity decreased in left eye
VA↓OU	visual acuity decreased in both eyes
VAR	visual-aural range
var	varicose, varicosities
var	variable, variation, varient, variometer, various, varying
VARO	Veteran's Administration Regional Office
vasc	vascular
vas vitr *vas vitreum*	a glass vessel
VAT	ventricular activation time
VBP	venous blood pressure
VC	ventricular contractions
VC	vital capacity
VC	color vision acuity
VC	voluntary closing
vc	vocal cord
V-C(ratio)	ventilation-circulation ratio
VCC	vasoconstrictor center
VCG	vector cardiogram
VCS	vasoconstrictor substance
VD	vasodilator
VD	venereal disease
VD	venous dilatation

VD *ventriculo dextro*	left ventricle
VD	ventrodorsal
vd	double vibrations
vd	void, voided (urinate)
VDC	vasodilator center
VDEL	Venereal Disease Experimental Laboratory
VDG	venereal disease, gonorrhea
vdg qs	voiding sufficient quantity
VDH	valvular disease of the heart
(no) VD or M	(no) venous distention or masses
VDM	vasodepressor material
VDRL	Venereal Disease Research Laboratory
VDS	vasodilator substance
VDS	venereal disease, syphilis
VE	esophageal lead (electrocardiogram)
VE	vaginal examination
VE	ventilatory equivalent (index)
VE	vesicular exanthema
V/E	vaginal examination
VEE	Venezuelan equine encephalomyelitis
vel, veloc	velocity
VEM	vasoexciter material
Ven, ven	venous
vent	ventilation

vent	ventral
vent	ventricle, ventricular
vent fib, ventric fib	ventricular fibrillation
ventric	ventricular
vert	vertebra
vert	vertical
vert	vertigo
vert comp, vert compr	vertical compression
vert comp, vert compr	vertebral compression
ves	vesicle, vesicular
ves *vesica*	bladder
ves	vessel
ves *vesicula*	blister
ves ur *vesica urinaria*	urinary bladder
V et *vide etiam*	see also
vet	veteran
Vet Adm	Veteran's Administration
V factor	verbal comprehension factor (psychiatry)
VF∗∗∗, VF∗∗∗	voluntary free breathing capacity at rate of choice of patient
VF	visual fields
VF	vocal fremitus
VFI	visual fields intact

VG	ventricular gallop
VG	very good
VG	volume of gas
VGRS	Vocational Guidance and Rehabilitation Service
VH	ventricular hypertrophy
VHF	very high frequency
VI	vaginal irrigation
VI	volume index
VIA	virus inactivating agent
VIB	Vocational Interest Blank
vib	vibration, vibratory
vibs	vocabulary, information, block design, similarities (psychiatry)
VIC	vasoinhibitory center
vic *vices*	times
vid *vide*	see
VIG	vaccine immune globulin
Vin *vinethene*	vinyl ether
vin *vinum*	wine
VIP	venereally infected person
vis *vide licet*	namely
vis	visible
vis	vision

vis	visiting, visitors
VISAB	Vocational Interest Scale for Adult Blind
visc	visceral
visc	viscous, viscosity
VISTA	Volunteers In Service To America
vit	vital
vit	vitamin
vit	vitreous (usually refers to vitreous body of the eye)
vit ov sol *vitello ovi solutas*	dissolved in yolk of egg
vit cap	vital capacity
vitel *vitellus*	yolk
vitr *vitreum*	glass
viz *vide licet*	namely
VJC	ventriculo-jugulo-cardiac shunt
VL	vision, left
VLF	very low frequency
VM	vasomotor
VM	vestibular membrane
VM	viomycin
VM	viscous metamorphosis
VM, vm	volt meter
VMA	vanillyl mandelic acid

VMC	vasomotor center
VMR	vasomotor rhinitis
VMS	visual memory span
VMT	vasomotor tone
VNA	Visiting Nurse Association
VNR	ventral nerve root
VO, V/O	verbal order
VO	voluntary opening
voc	vocation, vocational
vocab	vocabulary
VOD *vision oculus dexter*	vision right eye
vol	volar
vol	volatile
vol	volume, volumetric
vol	voluntary
vol	volunteer
Vol Adm	voluntary admission (psychiatric)
vol %	volume per cent
VOS *vision oculus sinister*	vision left eye
VOS *vitello ovi solutas*	dissolved in yolk of egg
VP	vapor pressure
VP	venous pressure
↓ VP	decreased venous pressure

↗ VP	increased venous pressure
VP	physiological volume
VP test	Vosges-Proskauer test
V-P ratio	ventilation-perfusion ratio
V ¢ P	vagotomy and pyloroplasty
VPB	ventricular premature beats
VPC	ventricular premature contractions
VPC	volume packed cells
VPS	vibrations per second
VQ	voice quality
VR	variable ratio
VR	venous return
VR	ventral root
VR	ventricular rate
VR	vision, right
VR	vocal resonance
VRA	Vocational Rehabilitation Administration Prior to 1963 this was the Office of Vocational Rehabilitation (OVR)
VRC	ventral nerve root, cervical
VRC_1, VRC_2, VRC_3, etc.	ventral root cervical by number
VRI	virus respiratory infection
VRL	ventral nerve root, lumbar
VRL_1, VRL_2, VRL_3, etc.	ventral root lumbar by number
VRMS	Van Riper memory span (auditory)
VRT	ventral nerve root, thoracic

VRT$_1$, VRT$_2$, VRT$_3$ etc.	ventral root, thoracic, by number
VRV	ventricular residual volume
VS	vesicular sounds (auscultation of chest)
VS	vital signs
VS	volumetric solution
Vs	venesection
vs *versus*	against
vs *vide supra*	see above
vs	vibration seconds
vs	single vibrations
vs, v/s	visited, visitors
VsB	venesection brachii
VSBE	very short below elbow
VSCT	ventral spinothalmic tract
VSD	ventricular septal defect (heart)
VSHD	ventricular septal heart defect
VST	ventral spinothalamic tract
V$^+$ substance	kyurenine
VT	vacuum tuberculin
VT	tetrazolium violet
VT	gas volume unit time
VT***	voluntary maximum breathing rate timed by metronome
V ⚡ T	volume and tension (pulse)

VTE	vicarious trial and error (psychiatry)
VTI	volume thickness index
Vtx	vertex presentation (obstetrics)
VV	vagina and vulva
VV, vv	varicose veins
vv *vice versa*	conversely
v/v	volume in volume percent
VV lig	varicose vein ligation
VW, vw	vessel wall

W	ward
W	water
W	watt
W	weak, weakness
W	white
W	wide, width
W	widow, widower
W	wolfram, tungsten
W	word fluency (psychiatry)
W	wound
W (response)	whole response
w	water
w	weak
w	white
w	wide, width
w	widow, widower
w, w/	with
w	wound
WA	wide awake (state of consciousness)
Wa, wa	when awake
wa	with average
W/A	white adult
W/a, W or A	weakness or atrophy
WAC	Women's Army Corps
WAF	weakness, atrophy, fasciculation

WAF	white adult female
WAIS	Wechsler's Adult Intelligence Scale
WAM	white adult male
WAR	Wasserman antigen reaction
Wass	Wasserman test (for syphilis)
WB	waist belt (restraint)
WB	washable base
WB	Wechsler-Bellevue Scale
WB	weight bearing
WB	westbound (position of car in accident)
WB	whole blood
Wb	Weber
WBC	well baby care
WBC	Well Baby Clinic
WBC	white blood cell, white blood corpuscle
WBC	white blood count
WBC diff	white blood count and differential
WBM	whole boiled milk
WBT	wet bulb temperature
WC	wheel chair
WC	white child
WC	will call
WC	wound check
W/C	watts per cubic centimeter
W/C	wheel chair

W
X
Y
Z

W/C	white child
wc	water closet (British and Canadian term for bathroom)
wc, w/c	wheel chair
wc	wound check
WCAB	Workman's Compensation Appeals Board
WD	well developed
WD	wet dressing
W/D	warm and dry
W/D	well developed
wd	ward
wd, w/d, w-d	well developed
wd	wound
WE, W/E	wound of entry
WEE	western equine encephalitis
wef	with effect from
*WF	West gas phase, fractional concentration
WF	wet films
WF	white female
WF	will follow
W/F	white female
wf	white female
WF-O	will follow in office
WH	walking heel (cast)
WH	well healed

WH	well hydrated (skin, mucous membrane)
wh	whisper
wh	white
wh ch	wheel chair
WHNS	well healed, non-symptomatic (wound)
WHO	World Health Organization
W hr	watt hour
wh/was	which was
WIA	wounded in action
Wid, wid	widow, widower
WISC	Wechsler Intelligence Scale for Children
WK disease	Wilson-Kimmelstiel disease
wk	weak
wk	week
wk	work
WL	waiting list
WL medium	Wallenstein laboratory medium
WL	wave length
WM, W/M	white male
WM	whole mount
wm	white male
Wm flex ex	Williams flexion exercises
WMO	Ward Medical Officer
WN, W/N	well nourished
wn, w/n, w-n	well nourished

WNL	within normal limits
WO	written order
W/O	will order
W/O	without
WOE	wound of entry
WOX	wound of exit
wpm	words per minute
WP	water packed
WP	wet pack
WP	whirlpool
WP	working point
WPB	whirlpool bath
WPES	Work and Personal Evaluation Services
WPW syndrome	Wolff-Parkinson-White syndrome
WR	Wasserman reaction
WR	weak response
W/S, ws	well supported (as abdomen or perineum)
WT	water temperature
WT	work therapy
wt	weight
wt b	weight bearing
WTC	Work Test Clinic
W/U	work up
W/V	weight by volume
W/wo	with or without

WWII

World War II – usually seen in combinations such as: SC WWII which means Service connected (injury or illness) World War II

W/X, w/x

wound of exit

X	cross
X	exposure
X	extremity
X	Kleinbock's unit (xray dosage)
X	magnification Example: 2 X = twice original size
X	ten (Roman numeral)
X	times (number of doses or treatments) Example: VS q 15 m X 4 = vital signs every 15 minutes four times
X	unknown factor, unknown quantity
X	xray
x	cross
x	exposure
x	extremity
x	unknown factor, unknown quantity
x	xanthine
x, Ⓧ	xray
Xa	chiasma
Xam	examination
X-Bein	genu valgum
X bodies	Bartonella baciliformis (bacteriology)
X chromosone	female sex chromosone
X disease	morbid symptoms of unknown origin
x'd	xrayed
Xe, xe	xenon

X element	the necessary chromosone
X factor	Christmas factor
X Hufte	coxa valga
X-ized	crystalized
X match, x match	cross match (blood for transfusion)
XOM	extra ocular movements
XOOP	xrays out of plaster
XOP	xrays out of plaster
X prep	xray preparation
xr	xray
x sect	cross section
XT	exotropia (measurement of squint)
X test	Xenopus test
Xta	chiasmata
Xtal	crystal
XU	excretory urogram
X walk	cross walk
XX	any expiratory gas
XYL, Xyl	xylocaine
Xyl ₵ cort	xylocaine and cortisone
X Zehe	halux valgus

Y	ordinate
Y, y	years
Y, y	young
Y	yttrium
Y/A	years ago, years of age
Y band	ileo-femoral band
Y chrom	male sex chromosone
yd	yard
YE	yellow enzyme
YEH_2	reduced yellow enzyme
yel	yellow
Y/O, y/o	years old
yr	year
YS, ys	yellow spot (on the retina)
Yt	yttrium
Z	atomic number
Z_1, Z_2, Z_3, etc	increasing degrees of contraction
Z	zero
Z	Zwichenscheibe intermediate disc
Z	Zuckung
z	standard score
z	zero
z	zone
Zn	zinc
Zr	zirconium
Zz	Zingiber

MEDICAL HIEROGLYPHS

Symbols

¢	and
∧	and
⌐	not
∨	or
*	supposed, presumed, not verified
?	possible, suggested, questionable
△	change
△	prism diopter (ophthalmology)
△	occipital triangle
⚡	triple arthrodesis
◇	eye
⬭	ptosis, lid lag
⬮	dilated pupil
[ ]	concentration

⌐	right upper quadrant	)
		) Areas indicated
⌐	right lower quadrant	) on patient while
		) he is facing the
⌐	left upper quadrant	) examiner
		)
⌐	left lower quadrant	)

⌐→	right turn (description of accident)
←⌐	left turn (description of accident)
□	male (rarely used)
/	virgule used to indicate either meaning Example: and/or

/	extension, extensor

/   fraction (divided by)
Examples: N/2 = ½ normal
               3/N = three times normal

/   organic

/   per
Example: 5 WBC/HPF = five white blood cells per high power field

/   to
Example: A/G ratio = albumin to globulin ratio

//   for

//   parallel, parallel bars

⌢   arc

~   similar cycle, cycle

~   about, approximately

≡   identical

≈   approximately identical

≢   not identical

⇕   equivalent to

⇕   not equivalent to

=   equal

≐ or ≈   approximately equal

≠   not equal

≤ or ≤   equal to or less than

≥ or ≥   equal to or greater than

≮   not less than

<   less than, smaller than, less severe than

$>$	greater than, larger than, more severe than, worse than
$\not>$	not greater than
$\angle$	angle
$\angle s$	angles
$\angle E$	angle of entry (bullet, missile, etc.)
$\angle x$	angle of exit
$\angle$	flexion, flexor
$\angle s$	flexors
✓	check, observe for
✓ 'd	checked, examined, observed
✓ g, ✓ ing	checking
✓	voided (urinary voiding)
✓ qs	voided sufficient quantity
⤺	voided and bowels moved
ṫ	bowel movement (The roman numeral indicates the number of stools in a given period if patient has diarrhea. Example: iii indicates three stools vi indicates six stools etc.
← or ⟨	proximal
← or ⟨	caused by, produced by, derived from
⇄	reversible reaction (chemical)
→ or ⟩	causes
→ or ⟩	demonstrates
→ or ⟩	distal
→ or ⟩	followed by
→ or ⟩	implies

→ or ⟩	indicates
→ or ⟩	leads to
→ or ⟩	produces
→ or ⟩	radiates to, radiating to
→ or ⟩	results in
→ or ⟩	reveals
→ or ⟩	shows
→ or ⟩	to, toward
→ or ⟩	yields
⇒	implies, implication
↔ or ⋀	width, widened
⟲	circumduction
⊙	encircling, girdling
↓ or ∨	below
↓ or ∨	decreased
↓ or ∨	deficiency, deficit
↓ or ∨	depressed
↓ or ∨	deteriorated, deteriorating
↓ or ∨	dimished, diminution
↓ or ∨	down
↓ or ∨	inferior
↓ or ∨	less than
↓ or ∨	low, lower

Examples: ↓ back = low back
             ↓ C sp area = lower cervical spine

| ↓ | precipitates |

↓g	decreasing, diminishing Example: Temperature ↓ = temperature dropping or decreasing
↓g	falling lowering Example: BP ↓ g = blood pressure falling
↓↓	down bilaterally Examples: testes ↓↓ = both testes descended plantar reflexes ↓↓ = plantar reflexes normal
↑↓	reversible reaction
↑↓	up and down
∧	and
↑ or ∧	above
↑ or ∧	elevated
↑ or ∧	enlarged
↑ or ∧	greater than
↑ or ∧	improved
↑ or ∧	increased
↑ or ∧	more than
↑ or ∧	superior (position)
↑ or ∧	upper
↗	deviated, displaced Example: ↗$_{10°}$ = deviation of 10 degrees
↑↑	positive Babinski
°	(temperature) degree Example: 99° R = 99 degree rectal temperature
°	(measurement) degree − 1/360 of a circle
°	(severity) degree − indicates severity of wounds or burns
Wounds-	1° = superficial 2° = moderate 3° = severe

Burns-	$1°$ = superficial, erythemal burn $2°$ = blistering $3°$ = destruction of epidermis and laying bare of sensitive nerve endings $4°$ = destruction of entire thickness of the skin and the subcutaneous connective tissue $5°$ = charring of the soft parts of the bone
$1°$, $2°$, $3°$, etc.	(time) one hour, two hours, etc.
$2°$	secondary to, due to, because of
′	primary accent
′	univalent
$1'$, $2'$, $3'$, etc.	(time) one hour, two hours, three hours, etc.
$1'$, $2'$, $3'$, etc.	(dimensions) one foot, two feet, etc.
″	bilavent
″	ditto
″	inch, inches Example: $2''$ = two inches
″	(time) minute (1/60 of an hour) Example: q $10''$ = every ten minutes
″	(measurement) second (1/60 of a degree)
″	secondary accent
‴	line (1/12 inch)
‴	trivalent
#	fracture
#	number
#	pound, pounds
$\sqrt{}$	root, radical
$\sqrt[2]{}$	square root
$\sqrt[3]{}$	cube root

%	per cent (number of parts per hundred parts)
:	ratio Example: 1:1000 solution
::	equality between ratios
1:1	one to one relationship (psychiatry)
∵	because, since
∴	therefore
...	no data (in a given category)
÷	divided by, division
⟋⟋⟋⟋⟋	rotation
∾	proportionate to
∝	variant, varies
∞	infinity, indefinitely more
∂	differential
●	bullet
☠	poison
☾ (Moon)	silver
♄ (Saturn)	lead
♃ (Jupiter)	tin
☿ (Mercury)	mercury
☉ (Sun)	gold
♂ (Mars)	iron
♂ (Mars)	male
♀ (Venus)	copper
♀ (Venus)	female

℞ (derived from ♃ Jupiter)	"take thou" used as a superscription for a prescription; used also to indicate any medication or treatment ordered
○	female (rarely used)
○	sex undetermined
□	male (rarely used)
*	birth
*	assumed, not verified
†	death, deceased
θ	temperature above zero degree Centigrade Example: 30 θ
0, θ, Ø	absent
0, θ, Ø	negative
0, θ, Ø	nil
0, θ, Ø	no, none
0, θ, Ø	without
L K } 0, θ, or Ø S	liver, kidneys, spleen negative (i.e. not palpable)
M T } 0, θ, or Ø R	no masses, tenderness or rebound (abdominal examination)
L M K Ø T S R	liver, kidneys and spleen not palpable and no masses, tenderness or rebound
—	absent
—	alkaline reaction
—	deficiency, deficient
—	minus
—	negative

—	nil
—	no, none
—	without
±	doubtful
±	either positive or negative
±	equivocal
±	indefinite
±	more or less
±	plus or minus
±	questionable
±	suggestive
±	variable
±	with or without
?	possible, doubtful, questionable
+	acid reaction
+	added to
+	and
+	excess
+	mild
+	plus (slightly more than stated amount)
+	positive
+	present
(+)ive	positive

Reflexes

0, 0̶, Ø	absent, negative
±, ?	questionable, flicker, equivocal
+	diminished, decreased, sluggish
++, ++̶, ‡	normally active
+++, +++̶	increased, moderately hyperactive
++++, ++++̶	markedly hyperactive
NT, nt	indicates not tested (usually because of obvious fracture, cast, hemiplegia, etc.)

Occasionally a doctor will use + or x to indicate the reflexes tested then write the findings beside the figure

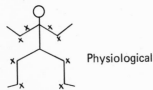

Physiological

Designation of severity (pain, spasm, tenderness, tightness, etc.)

0, 0̶, Ø	negative
±	very slight
+	mild
±±	mild to moderate
++, ++̶, ‡	moderate
+++, +++̶	moderately severe
++++, ++++̶	markedly severe pain: spastic muscles
?	doubtful, questionable, possible, suggestive, not tested
NT	not tested

Evaluation of pain and related disability

± to +   *Minimal* pain causes annoyance but no handicap

+ to ±±   *Slight* pain can be tolerated but causes some handicap in performance of activities which precipitate pain

++, ⧺   *Moderate* pain can be tolerated for short periods of time but causes handicap in performance of the activities which precipitate pain

+++, ⧻   *Moderately severe* pain causes handicap in the performance of activities which precipitate pain

++++, ⧼   *Severe* pain precludes any activity which precipitates the pain and may be completely disabling

Qualitative tests

0, θ, ∅   negative

±   very slight trace, equivocal

+   slight trace (noticeable reaction)

++, ++   trace

+++, +++   moderate reaction

++++, ++++   large amount, pronounced reaction

Wasserman test results

+   less than 50% inhibition of hemolysis

++   50% inhibition of hemolysis

+++   75% inhibition of hemolysis

++++   complete inhibition of hemolysis

Amounts, dosages, etc.

Roman numerals are used frequently. They are usually written in lower case with a dot above each i, to avoid the possibility of confusing a carelessly written ı∕ for a ∨. Handwritten numbers are usually written with a line above the ones and the dots above the line.

Examples: i, ii, iii, iv, v, vi, vii, viii, ix, x

$\dot{\overline{i}}, \overline{i\dot{i}}, \overline{i\dot{i}\dot{i}}, \overline{iv}, \overline{v}, \overline{vi}, \overline{vi\dot{i}}, \overline{vii\dot{i}}, \overline{i\dot{x}}, x$

The decimal system is used frequently and the position of the decimal point is emphasized by the use of zero.

Examples: 0.5 gm = 5/10th gram

5.0 gm = 5 grams (ten times as large a dose as the dose above)

Amounts are stressed by writing drams, grams, grains, etc. before the numeral.

Examples: gr iss = one and a half grains

ℨ ii = drams two

ℨ	dram
℥	ounce
℈	scruple
flℨ, fld ℨ	fluid dram
fl℥, fld ℥	fluid ounce

Blood clotting factors

Factor I	fibrinogen
Factor II	prothrombin
Factor III	tissue thromboplastin
Factor IV	calcium
Factor V	prothrombokinase
Factor VI	(still controversial)
Factor VII	serum prothrombin conversion accelerator
Factor VIII	antihemophilic globulin A
Factor IX	plasma thromboplastin component (Christmas factor)

Factor X	Stuart-Prower factor (required for prothrombin conversion)
Factor XI	plasma thromboplastin antecedent
Factor XII	Hageman factor — deficiency results in great prolongation of clotting time of venous blood
4 arm	forearm
Fig 4	figure four test (Fabere test)

English letters used as symbols

@	at
āā *ana*	of each, equal parts
A°, Å	Angstrom unit
C′	complement
°C	Centigrade (degrees)
c̄, c̄, ċ *cum*	with
E。	electroaffinity
¢ *et*	and
ⓔⓐ	each
°F	Farenheit (degrees)
f ℥, fld ℥	fluid dram
f ℥, fld ℥	fluid ounce
f	frequency
ƒ	function
/ƒ/	function
Ⓗ , ⓗ	hypodermic
ⓘⓜ	intramuscular

Ⓘⓥ	intravenous
Ⓛ	left
ⓜ	by mouth
ⓜ	murmur
ᵥⓜ	factitial murmur
M	minim
~~M~~	mix
$\aleph$P, $\diagup$P	high energy phosphate bond
○	female
O, $\overline{O}$ *octarius*	pint
⊙	oral, orally
O_2	oxygen
QO_2	oxygen consumption
®	rectal
®	right
$\bar{\dot{s}}$, $\bar{s}$, $\dot{s}$ *sine*	without
$\bar{\dot{s}}\bar{\dot{s}}$, $\bar{s}\bar{s}$, $\dot{s}\dot{s}$ *semis*	half
X, x	by (in statement of dimensions) Example: 3 cm x 2 cm
X, x	cross Example: Xmatch iiU WB = cross match two units whole blood
X, x	score
X, x	times (symbol of magnification or multiplication)
X, x	times (repetitions − indication of the number of doses or number of treatments ordered) Examples: X i = one time only X iii = 3 doses or 3 treatments

$\bar{X}$ mean of sample observations

2 x 2)   gauze dressings which have been folded to these
4 x 4)   dimensions
4 x 8)

Methods of administering medications

clysis   hypodermoclysis

Ⓗ , ⓗ   hypodermic, hypodermically

Ⓜ   intramuscularly

Ⓥ   intravenously

ⓜ   by mouth

Ⓞ   orally

Ⓡ   rectally

Temperature taken by

Ⓐ , ⓐₓ   axilla

ⓜ   mouth

Ⓡ   rectum

Greek letters and combinations with greek letters

α (lower case alpha)   in proportion to

β (lower case beta)   Chemistry 1) Used to indicate the substitution
                                                        of a hydrogen atom at the second
                                                        carbon atom from a functional group
                                                        2) The second in a series of isomeric
                                                        compounds

γ (lower case gamma)   gamma
                                               Example: globulin = gamma globulin

Δ (upper case delta)   Anatomy — a triangular surface
                                               Chemistry 1) position of unsaturated linkage
                                                        (double bond)

Δ (upper case delta)

2) an atom grouping located on the fourth carbon from the carboxyl group or other functional group
3) fourth in a series of compounds

η (lower case eta)   viscosity

κ (lower case kappa)   symbol for the 10th carbon atom

λ (lower case lambda)   wavelength

μ (lower case mu)   micro

μ (lower case mu)   symbol of a linear measurement, micron, micrometer (one millionth of a meter or one thousandth of a millimeter)

μ (lower case mu)   modulus

μa   microampere

μc   microcurie

μf   microfarad

μμg, μμgm   micromicrogram

μl   microliter

μm   micromole

μμ   micromicron

μOsm   microosmol

μr   microroentgen

μs   microsecond

μv   microvolt

μw   microwatt

π (lower case pi)   osmotic pressure

Σ (upper case sigma)   summation, sum of

Σ (upper case sigma)   sum of frequency deviation

σ (lower case sigma)	millisecond (1/1000 second)
σ (lower case sigma)	standard deviation
Ψ ψ (upper or lower case psi)	psychology
Ω (upper case omega)	ohm

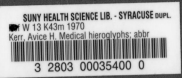
3/18/2010
Retain

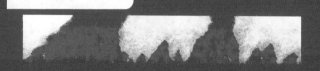